‖‖ ‖ ‖‖‖‖‖‖‖‖‖‖‖‖‖‖‖‖‖‖‖‖‖‖‖‖‖ ‖‖‖ ‖‖ ‖‖

✔ **KU-331-544**

Working with Interpreters in Mental Health

In today's society, there is an increasing need for mental health professionals to work with interpreters, yet coverage of this subject in the existing literature is scarce. *Working with Interpreters in Mental Health* gives an insight into the issues and challenges facing professionals working with interpreters.

Informed by theoretical, research and practice considerations, *Working with Interpreters in Mental Health* helps practitioners to develop better ways of helping service users who need an interpreter. Combining contributions from a number of different disciplines, this book discusses:

- Interpreters in medical consultations
- Issues of language provision in health care services
- The application of theoretical frameworks to the work with interpreters
- The work of interpreters in a variety of practical settings

Whilst the focus is placed within a mental health context, many of the issues raised apply equally to other contexts where interpreters are needed. This book will be invaluable for practitioners of psychology, psychiatry, nursing, social work and allied health care professionals.

Rachel Tribe is senior lecturer in Psychology at the University of East London. She has many years' experience of working with clients from different cultural and racial backgrounds in mental health settings, and has a particular interest in the area of the refugee context of mental health.

Hitesh Raval is a clinical psychologist and systemic family psychotherapist, currently working as a clinical research director at Salomons in Tunbridge Wells, Kent. He has also been substantially involved in the training of clinical psychologists and systemic family psychotherapists.

HS 362.2 TRIB

Working with Interpreters in Mental Health

Edited by Rachel Tribe and Hitesh Raval

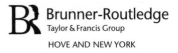

Brunner-Routledge
Taylor & Francis Group

HOVE AND NEW YORK

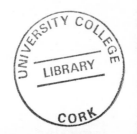

i 166 14197

First published 2003 by Brunner-Routledge
27 Church Road, Hove, East Sussex, BN3 2FA

Simultaneously published in the USA and Canada
by Brunner-Routledge
29 West 35th Street, New York, NY 10001

Brunner-Routledge is an imprint of the Taylor & Francis Group

© 2002 Edited by Rachel Tribe and Hitesh Raval

Paperback cover design by Sandra Heath
Typeset in Times by Mayhew Typesetting, Rhayader, Powys
Printed and bound in Great Britain by TJ International Ltd,
Padstow, Cornwall

All rights reserved. No part of this book may be reprinted or reproduced
or utilised in any form or by any electronic, mechanical, or other means,
now known or hereafter invented, including photocopying and recording,
or in any information storage or retrieval system, without permission in
writing from the publishers.

British Library Cataloguing in Publication Data
A catalogue record for this book is available from the British Library

Library of Congress Cataloging-in-Publication Data
Working with interpreters in mental health / edited by Rachel Tribe and
Hitesh Raval.
      p. cm.
   Includes bibliographical references and index.
   ISBN 0-415-18878-4 (hbk) – ISBN 0-415-18879-2 (pbk.)
     1. Mental health services–Great Britain. 2. Translators–Great
Britain. I. Tribe, Rachel. II. Raval, Hitesh.

   RA790.7.G7 W674 2002
   362.2'0941–dc21

                                                          2002071244

ISBN 0-415-18878-4 (hbk)
ISBN 0-415-18879-2 (pbk)

Contents

List of contributors   vii
Acknowledgements   xii
Tribute to Maxwell Mudarikiri   xiii

Introduction   1
RACHEL TRIBE AND HITESH RAVAL

1 An overview of the issues in the work with
interpreters   8
HITESH RAVAL

2 Interpreters in medical consultations   30
ANNIE CUSHING

3 Training issues for interpreters   54
RACHEL TRIBE WITH MARSHA SANDERS

4 Issues of language provision in health care services   69
AKGUL BAYLAV

5 A day in the life of an interpreting service   77
FARDIS NIJAD

6 An interpreter's perspective   92
MINOO RAZBAN

7 The role and experience of interpreters   99
EMILY GRANGER AND MARTYN BAKER

8 Applying theoretical frameworks to the work with
   interpreters   122
   HITESH RAVAL

9 From postmen to makers of meaning: a model for
   collaborative work between clinicians and interpreters   135
   PHILIP MESSENT

10 The role of the interpreter in child mental health: the
   changing landscape   151
   ROSEMARY LOSHAK

11 Working with interpreters within services for people
   with learning disabilities.   168
   JOHN NEWLAND

12 Working with the interpreters in adult mental health   182
   MAXWELL MAGONDO MUDARIKIRI

13 The refugee context and the role of interpreters   198
   RACHEL TRIBE AND JEAN MORRISSEY

14 Speaking with the silent: addressing issues of
   disempowerment when working with refugee people   219
   NIMISHA PATEL

15 Narratives of translating–interpreting with refugees:
   the subjugation of individual discourses   238
   RENOS K. PAPADOPOULOS

16 Concluding comments   256
   RACHEL TRIBE AND HITESH RAVAL

Index   261

Contributors

Martyn Baker is a clinical psychologist and Academic Tutor at the University of East London. He has many years of clinical experience of working with clients from diverse minority ethnic backgrounds, as well as being an experienced trainer of clinical psychologists.

Akgul Baylay trained as a psychologist to PhD level and worked as a university lecturer and researcher in Turkey. She has been involved in various aspects of bilingual community work in the UK, with particular interest in health interpreting and bilingual health advocacy since 1983. She is currently employed as the qualities manager at East London and City Health authority and has worked in the NHS since 1983, setting up, managing and developing bilingual services to support the black and ethnic communities in London. She has written a number of articles about communication and access to health services in the medical and social press, including a Special Report published in *The Practitioner*.

Annie Cushing is a senior lecturer and communication skills co-ordinator at St Bartholemew's and the Royal London Hospital School of Medicine and Dentistry. With many years of clinical and education experience as a dentist in teaching hospitals and the community, her interest in the influence of the professional–patient relationship in health care led her into the field of inter-personal and communication skills education. She has devised innovative assessments based on learners' developing insights into their own skills and learning needs, and has contributed to international conferences on medical education. She has introduced sessions in the undergraduate curriculum for medical and dental students on cross-cultural communication and the role of health advocates.

Emily Granger is a clinical psychologist working with children and families, who developed an interest in working with interpreters during her pre-qualification training in clinical psychology. She converted this interest into an innovative research project giving interpreters a chance to voice their experiences of carrying out their work.

Rosemary Loshak is an experienced psychiatric social worker who has used her strong interests in psychoanalytic approaches, parental mental illness and multicultural work in thinking about her work with interpreters. She has extensive experience of working as a social worker in an inner London child and adolescent mental health team serving a multicultural local community. She has been the driving force of what was a unique service at the time when it was set up, of employing and training up interpreters based specifically in the child and adolescent mental health service.

Maxwell Magondo Mudarikiri migrated to Britain from Zimbabwe where he worked in the public medical health care setting, specialising in HIV/AIDS work. He was a British trained systemic family psychotherapist, who worked as a trainer of systemic family psychotherapists. He also worked in adult mental health settings as a practitioner in London, where he carried out direct clinical work. He provided supervision to counsellors and consultation to organisations.

Jean Morrissey works at the Nethersole School of Nursing, Chinese University of Hong Kong. She has lived and worked in several countries and has many years' experience of working with a diverse range of ethnic groups. She started her career as a nurse and more recently has worked as a trainer, university lecturer, consultant, supervisor and therapist. She has been published on the subject of clinical supervision.

Philip Messent is an experienced social worker and systemic family psychotherapist who has developed his extensive clinical practice in an inner London child and adolescent mental health service, in a strongly multicultural local population work context. He is also a trainer on systemic family psychotherapy courses, and brings his systemic insights into his work with interpreters. Since 1986, he has been employed as a Child Mental Health Social Work Team Manager by the London Borough of Tower Hamlets and is based at the Emmanuel Miller Centre, Gill St, E14.

John Newland is a Chartered Clinical Psychologist. He has worked for over 10 years in the multicultural London Borough of Islington. He has a strong interest in promoting inclusive thinking and practice for black and minority ethnic people with learning disabilities. Within the Division of Clinical Psychology, he held the post of elected Chair of the 'Race' & Culture Special Interest Group from 1994 to 1998. His published work focuses on understanding ethnic identity. He is a visiting lecturer to numerous Clinical Psychology training courses.

Fardis Nijad is director and founder of Essential Interpreters and Translators International (EITI), 295–297 High Street, Slough, S11 1BD. EITI employs over 800 professionals in over 100 languages as well as 8 full-time staff. His duties include market research, business planning and strategy, recruitment, interpreter and user training, and skill evaluation. He is a member of FRES (Federation of Recruitment and Employment Services). In addition Fardis has experience of working as an interpreter and researcher in Greece and various parts of the USA.

Renos K. Papadopoulos is Professor of Analytic Psychology at the Centre for Psychoanalytic Studies at the University of Essex, Consultant Clinical Psychologist and Systemic Family Psychotherapist at the Tavistock Clinic, and is a training and supervising Jungian psychoanalyst practicing in London. He has an extensive publication record. His last two books are *Multiple Voices-Narrative in Systemic Psychotherapy* (co-edited with John Byng-Hall) and the four volume edited collection of essays entitled *C.G. Jung: Critical Assessments*. He is editor of *Harvest Journal for Jungian Studies*, and he is Chairman of the Academic Standing Subcommittee of the International Association for Analytical Psychology. As a consultant to the United Nations and other organisations, he has worked with survivors of violence and disaster in several countries.

Nimisha Patel is a senior lecturer in clinical psychology at the University of East London and a consultant clinical psychologist, and Head of clinical psychology at the Medical Foundation caring for victims of torture. She has also worked for many years in the NHS as a practitioner/clinician, researcher and in developing clinical practice and services for a multi-ethnic population. She has been published widely on issues of working with difference and discrimination in psychological health services.

Hitesh Raval is a clinical psychologist and systemic family psychotherapist. He has worked as a practitioner in child and adolescent mental health services, as well as working in academic settings providing pre-qualifying training for clinical psychologists and systemic family psychotherapists. He has substantial experience of working with families from different cultural groups, within a variety of different socio-economic contexts and work settings. His clinical and research interests are informed by multicultural considerations, and he has been published in this area of work. Currently he is working as a Clinical Research Director on the Salomon's clinical psychology training scheme.

Minoo Razban immigrated to Britain from the Middle East where she trained as an architect. She continued to work in this field following migration and parallel to this began working as an interpreter and translator. She is a registered Public Service Interpreter, and works in a number of health care, medico-legal and scientific work settings that require an interpreter or translator. She has a particular interest in the social dimension to mental health.

Marsha Sanders has worked for several years in the field of language support services, developing interpreting and translation facilities, and policy for public service users and providers who do not share a common language. She worked for several years as a research and development worker for an innovative language support project in London, which produced a directory of community interpreting services, and a handbook on interpreting and translation. She has also worked closely with a number of Local Authorities and NHS units to develop and support language mediation facilities, as well as developing partnerships with similar European projects, advising them in their first stages of setting up. More recently she has worked with homeless projects and in the health care setting, where she has developed a language and communication policy for one health authority, and has done consultancy work for several others, looking at a variety of equal access issues. She has been published in the area of interpreting.

Rachel Tribe is a senior lecturer, chartered psychologist and course director in the School of Psychology at the University of East London. She is an experienced clinician who has extensive experience of working with different cultural, racial and religious groups in the UK and other countries. Her work has involved consultancy to individual clients and teams as well as the evaluation of programmes on behalf of a range of organisations. She has also undertaken substantial training and organisational development work. She has had a number of academic articles published and presented papers at international conferences in the area of using interpreters and bicultural workers in mental health, as well as publishing articles in other related areas.

Acknowledgements

Hitesh Raval would like to thank the interpreters, clinicians and the families that he has worked with, who have each in their own way continued to keep alive the issue of interpreting for him. He would like to dedicate this book to Maya.

Rachel Tribe would like to thank all the interpreters that she has worked alongside in the UK and abroad, who have given so generously of their time in explaining cultural and political context, symbols, meanings, and language to her, particularly Chandra, Gameela, and Rane. She would like to dedicate this book to Prue and Ken, with thanks for everything.

Tribute to Maxwell Mudarikiri

Maxwell was a very experienced family therapy trainer. He always brought his liveliness, enthusiasm, thoughtfulness, spirituality and sensitivity to his encounters with his colleagues, those in training with him, and the families that he worked with in his clinical practice. Maxwell's particular style of working within a narrative family therapy approach was complementary to his ability to understand human suffering from different perspectives; in ways that also freed up others to be able to stand back and discover for themselves new insights and solutions to 'old problems'. In his gentle and thoughtful manner he was able to challenge discriminatory practices and the processes associated with them, and empower others to be able to do so in their own ways.

When discussing the initial idea for this book Maxwell was generous with both his support and commitment to the project. His immediate support for the idea and his willingness to contribute to this book was of immense help, and he was able to provide the much needed reassurance and belief that this project was worthwhile at the time when this was most needed. Maxwell has brought his unique and insightful way of grappling with the issues of working with interpreters to his chapter. His chapter also reflects his particular therapeutic approach and how he was able to adapt it in thinking about his work with interpreters. Through the different stages of this project Maxwell was a constant supportive force.

In this time of sorrow at his death there is no doubt that his spirit will remain with us. It is with sadness that we lost Maxwell before this particular project had come to fruition, as he would have been very proud of it. However, his presence remains in force through the thoughts and words that he has shared with us so generously in writing his chapter.

For those of us who were lucky to have known Maxwell, our conversations with him continue to guide our journeys, and those of the families that we work with, to landscapes and places that Maxwell had not only made imaginable but also possible to find in this physical existence that we call 'life'.

Hitesh Raval

Introduction

Rachel Tribe and Hitesh Raval

The idea for this book came out of the authors' concern that such a book did not already exist and from the realisation in our own clinical experiences that there was a need for information about working with interpreters. We were surprised to find that work with interpreters has had very little representation in journals or books.

While understanding and knowledge of practice-based interpreting within mental health appears to be expanding, it seems that this has not been reflected by a concomitant increase in published material. This may have the undesirable effect that knowledge gained in one area of specialism or geographical location cannot easily be accessed, shared, or further developed by others working in different contexts or locations. We hope this book may go some way towards bridging these gaps and stimulating further discussion, debate and research in this important area. The lack of published work appears to be a missed opportunity given that many service users in Britain today are primary speakers of languages other than English. In addition statistical evidence shows that increasing numbers of people move across national boundaries throughout their lives. This may mean that groups of people are not able to access mental health services easily and they may receive a secondary service when they do, and that their contribution to mental health debates may be lost. There may be a number of reasons why there is not more published research and this book is an attempt to try and share knowledge and understanding and open up the debate.

Many service providers in health have responded to some extent to the need of their clients by making use of both trained and untrained interpreters. We include therefore one set of general briefing guidelines on working with interpreters (see p. 65). However, they were developed within one particular context and may require some fine-tuning if they are to be used in another.

This book is aimed at a wide readership, but particularly at people working in mental health, either with, or as, interpreters. Many of the issues will also have resonance for those working in other areas of health, but there are particular issues relating to the area of mental health that we believe require special consideration. We hope that the book may be useful to interpreters, managers with policy and service planning responsibilities, those in training who may need to work with interpreters in the future, and for those working in clinical, community, primary care or forensic settings. The chapters in this book mirror the wider debates within the arena of interpretation and mental health.

The contributors to this book are all experienced practitioners in the areas about which they have written, and come from a range of professions and positions, including interpreter, academic, manager, founder of an interpreting agency providing services to a range of organisations, psychologist, social worker, family therapist, advocate, and trainer among others.

Many of the chapters are clearly about clinical practice; others are personal accounts; and some are written from a more theoretical perspective. We believe that the different perspectives inform one another and add to our understanding of a range of issues within working with interpreters in mental health.

We are aware of one area, which we would have liked to have included in this book, but unfortunately we could not find anyone to write about interpreting within the area of mental health when working with deaf clients and we believe this is an unfortunate omission. In addition we have not included anything about the use of psychometric tests across languages and the interpretation of assessment instruments.

We have structured the book into broadly two sections in attempting to cover a number of professional and practice issues that may need to be considered when working with interpreters. The first section will look at professional issues in working with interpreters, and issues arising for interpreters in carrying out their work. One theme that is prominent in the first section is the lack of a professional identity and role frequently experienced by interpreters and those working alongside them. The theme is taken up by a number of authors in this book noticeably Baylav, Raval,

Nijad, Razban, Granger and Baker. This is an important debate within the area of mental health and interpreting. It is one that requires careful consideration if we are to ensure that access to mental health services is not limited to those speaking good English, as well as ensuring that different cultural perspectives are encouraged and represented in mental health debates and services.

The issue of training is another important area where both mental health workers and interpreters may benefit from training in working together. A training course curriculum might include such issues as models of interpreting, ethics, professional boundaries and responsibilities, logistics, and developing relationships and confidence in working both with and as an interpreter. Ensuring that communication channels remain open is vital so that different cultural beliefs about mental health can be heard and discussed by all parties. An understanding of mental health issues, whether diagnosis, treatment, underlying theory, or different ways of working and the importance of understanding cultural factors, should form an important part of any training programme. Granger and Baker, Nijad, Tribe with Saunders, and Baylav discuss the issue of the training of interpreters more fully in their chapters. We believe that ongoing debates around these issues can enhance clinical practice, and regular meetings where interpreters and clinicians meet to discuss relevant issues may prove to be time usefully spent.

Models of clinical practice are then looked at in the second section of the book. It is important to realise that there is not one sole accepted way of working with interpreters, as the situation, client's and clinician's requirements, the nature of the work and practice of the agency may all help determine this. The issue of what is meant by interpreting has been written about by many of the authors in this book and the various forms of interpreting remain one of the central debates within this book. It appears that there is no right or wrong answer, no 'one size fits all'. However, there is a need for those working as interpreters and the health professionals that work with them to be aware of the different possibilities and to take time to consider which is the most appropriate in each case. Including the interpreter in discussions before and after the session will assist the decision about this. For example, it may be that on occasions it is useful for the interpreter to translate verbatim, but on others it may be useful for the interpreter to act as a cultural consultant and explain cultural or health beliefs, as without these the consultation may be missing an important component. Also any regular clinical meetings held at the agency might wish to include issues of working with interpreters and ensuring that different cultural views are incorporated into clinical discussions, formulations and practice.

A large percentage of the contributors have experience of working both as interpreters and with interpreters and have drawn on these experiences in their chapters. There are likely to be both challenges and opportunities involved in using interpreters within mental health; these are discussed in more detail in the chapters of Mudarikiri, Patel and Messent. Working with interpreters has been described in some of the literature as making work more difficult. We acknowledge that on occasions working with interpreters may be challenging but also think that the different perspectives it brings to the work and the way it may lead to assumptions being questioned can only improve our practice and hopefully the whole debate. The authors have described a range of dilemmas that may occur when working with interpreters and we have tried where possible to offer solutions to some of these dilemmas. The specific issues relating to working with interpreters in the particular context of refugee service users are addressed in the penultimate three chapters; time and space constraints prevented us from covering more situations.

In summary the chapters cover the following areas. The first chapter, by Raval, offers an overview of the general issues to be found within the area of working with interpreters in mental health. The second chapter, by Annie Cushing, a clinician working in primary care, moves on to look at the kinds of issues which may arise when working in any primary care setting, and which we hope provides a useful general and practical introduction to working with interpreters. The third chapter, by Tribe with Saunders, addresses issues relating to training of interpreters and clinicians. Akgul Baylav (Chapter Four) writes of the service delivery issues encountered in the use of interpreters in the NHS in East London and makes some suggestions about how these may be overcome in innovative and different ways. As someone who has been involved in the provision of interpreting services for many years, she is able to draw on her own experiences. She recounts instances when clients have not been able to access health services, have relied on family members, including sometimes children, to interpret for them, or have used community workers. The latter group she notes may be excellent community workers, but may be untrained as interpreters or may lack the specialist vocabulary. She also writes of the need for service specifications or purchasing tools, which are based on a needs analysis where it has been decided what are the most appropriate for the type of language support services. She informs us that most health authorities in London have included elements of specifying language support services within their general quality specification. She also describes the process whereby some boroughs have found that holding dedicated sessions where language support is available improves the take up rate of services. Dedicated interpreting time can also be used to produce health promotion materials. She hypothesises that these sessions may improve better compliance with medication regimes, fewer errors in history-taking and better diagnosis, and that these sessions may therefore be cost-effective.

Fardis Nijad's chapter (Chapter Five) is based on his many years' working as an interpreter and also running an interpreting services agency. He raises important issues about the difficulties interpreters face when wanting to assist people with whom they share a language. He also writes about their difficulties when they cannot be guaranteed work and their subsequent problems with the taxation and welfare systems. His 'day in the life' chapter raises issues relating to service provision in an interesting and accessible way.

Minoo Razban's very personal account of her experiences of working as an interpreter gives us much to think about in Chapter Six. She makes the same point as Fardis Nijad that people employing interpreters may assume that all speakers of that language will understand a particular language. Unfortunately the use of dialect and specific words in each country or the integration of words from another language may mean that the two speakers cannot really communicate. This has particular resonance in the area of mental health. She also raises the important point of cultural taboos around mental health, for example, some people may fear others knowing that they have consulted a mental health professional or are seen as having a 'mental health problem'. She cites examples of when people have kept their difficulties hidden rather than expose them by seeking help. She also raises the issue of expectations that a patient may have of a mental health professional being able to sort out housing or welfare problems immediately, not understanding that in a segmented system this may not be possible or within the remit of the clinician.

The empirical study undertaken by Granger and Baker (Chapter Seven) appears to be one of the first, if not the first, pieces of research conducted in the UK to look at the role of interpreters from their own perspective, and to have some nomothetic data adds a useful element to the literature. Much of the current research literature has been based on idiographic/case study type data. The research participants represent a good sample of people working as paid interpreters in a range of languages. Some of the quotes given by the participants are extremely interesting and add a very useful and sometimes missing dimension to the debate. It is sobering to note in Granger and Baker's study that they found that 64 per cent of the interpreters were willing to change their job and only 50 per cent of them reported feeling valued by the professionals they worked alongside.

The second section of the book focuses on therapeutic work with interpreters, and theoretical models that help with developing this practice. Raval (Chapter Eight) summarises some theoretical frameworks that help us think about the work with interpreters, and reflects on how these frameworks can be applied to this work. The chapters that follow this draw to a greater or lesser extent on these frameworks when describing therapeutic work across different types of service contexts.

Philip Messent, a social worker/family therapist working in East London, writes in Chapter Nine of his own experiences in clinical practice and about the issues/need for an interpreter to move beyond the spoken word. He gives some excellent clinical examples of working as a team with an interpreter who obviously has a far better understanding of cultural variables, and of the interpreter's role in locating the client's emotional issues within their cultural and religious context. Messent writes about how an interpreter was far better placed to assist one client with an important psychosocial issue in relation to finding work in a new country. He also writes of the importance of using the resources within the therapeutic setting, rather than the clinician acting as the expert and casting the interpreter in the role of a mere interpreter of words.

In Chapter Ten Rosie Loshak goes on to write of her experiences of working with interpreters in her work with mainly Bangladeshi children. The clinical examples she gives are very pertinent and thought provoking. In Chapter Eleven John Newland writes of some of the dilemmas he experienced in working in the area of learning difficulties with clients, their families, and interpreters.

This is a very new area in which there is very little that has been published and the thinking and development of the theory is still in its infancy. However, he raises a number of very interesting questions about the subject and starts to consider some possible theoretical underpinnings.

Mudarikiri, in Chapter Twelve, uses social constructionism as his lens when viewing the issues related to working with interpreters. He notes the importance of viewing the positive contributions that interpreters can make in improving our understanding of cultural assumptions and health.

The final three chapters in this book focus more specifically on working with refugee service users. In Chapter Thirteen Rachel Tribe writes about interpreters and mental health with particular reference to refugees and the associated issues. This is followed by Nimisha Patel's chapter, in which she offers some important and challenging views relating to the ways interpreters have been used. She is again writing about working with refugees, but many of her points, for example her model of working with interpreters, might also be considered when working with other groups. Renos Papadopoulos in Chapter Fifteen offers some interesting views about the interaction between 'life and language' when working with a specific group of refugees. It is, however, important to note that some of the issues raised are likely to be specific to this group of Bosnian refugees. He raises some issues about the triangulation process that often occurs when one of the participants in the clinical triad does not share a language.

In summary, there needs to be much more research undertaken in this important area of working with interpreters in mental health. Models and service provision need to be developed which consider these issues as a matter of course. Perhaps most important is the point that language does not exist in isolation but is located within a socio-cultural and political context. Within a multicultural society different beliefs and views about mental health and the ways these are expressed need to be considered as a matter of course rather than as an add-on extra.

Chapter 1

An overview of the issues in the work with interpreters

Hitesh Raval

Introduction

Working with interpreters in health care settings can be challenging, enjoyable and demanding. In Britain there is no mandatory requirement on interpreters, or health care practitioners, to undertake any accredited training for carrying out clinical or therapeutic work (e.g. therapy, medical consultation, social work intervention), where language translation is required. Not many empirical studies have been conducted in this area of work. The limited literature on health care interpreting consists predominantly of accounts describing the difficulties that arise in this work. Also, there is an absence of a theoretical foundation underpinning clinical practice utilising interpreters.

This introductory chapter deals with several aspects related to clinical work utilising interpreters. First, some of the issues surrounding the provision of mental health services for people from ethnic minorities are briefly discussed. The need for interpreters is then addressed. The next section deals with the area of training for interpreters and health care practitioners. The work roles taken on by interpreters are also explored, and the experiences of interpreters, service users, and health care practitioners are reviewed. Ethical considerations in relation to the work of interpreters, and guidelines of good clinical practice are also thought about. The word 'clinician' is used in a generic manner to refer to mental health or medical practitioners.

Mental health provision for people from ethnic minorities

One of the consistent criticisms levelled at mental health provision in Britain is that it is still failing to provide culturally appropriate and equitable services to people from ethnic minorities (Fernando, 1995; Patel et al, 2000). This situation is not unique to Britain and is similar in other countries such as Canada and South Africa (Crawford, 1994; O'Neil et al, 1993). Mental health care provision in these countries is mainly resourced by personnel from the dominant white indigenous population, who are drawing on models of health care based on western cultural values. Health care practices based on non-western cultural traditions are given less importance or credence in mainstream medicine and mental health work. For example, standard texts in child clinical psychology (Herbert, 1991) and child psychiatry (Goodman and Scott, 1997; Rutter and Hersov, 1985) give almost no mention of culture.

There is restricted access to mental health care provision for many people of minority status. Restricted access often results from people not having sufficient information about how to seek out health care. Unwarranted myths, taboos, and stigmas, as well as justifiable beliefs about mental health services that are held by referrers or ethnic minority service users may act as barriers to seeking out appropriate services. Not speaking the dominant language of the host country becomes another barrier in gaining access to services. On gaining access ethnic minority service users may be confronted with a hostile and unfamiliar health care system. The services they encounter may expose them to further experiences of institutional racism, and culturally insensitive or inappropriate delivery of health care (Aitken, 1998; Fernando, 1995; Kaufert et al, 1985). Failure by mental health practitioners to address racism and normalising the inequalities in health care arising out of it, can further serve to make institutional racism invisible and thus allow discriminatory institutional practices to go unchallenged (Aitken, 1998; Drennan, 1999; Wetherell and Potter, 1992). Mental health practitioners, or clinicians who find it difficult to raise issues related to power and racism in an appropriate manner, may unwittingly subject the service user to further experiences of disempowerment and racism within the intimacy of the therapeutic consultation (Aitken, 1998; Ridley, 1995). An individual user's experience of mental health services will also be influenced by how issues related to difference are negotiated with the clinician, and the manner in which an understanding of the user's difficulties is brought about.

Factors influencing the type of service delivery

In meeting the needs of a service user through an affirming therapeutic relationship, the clinician has to take into account issues related to power and the wider context (Smail, 1990). Clinicians hold greater power in relation to service users by virtue of their specialist professional knowledge and the technical language that goes with it. The power differential and inequality between the clinician and the service user becomes greater when there are differences in language and culture, and the service user is disadvantaged by not being able to speak the dominant language of the host country.

The quality and type of service provision in any one setting is influenced by the broader and local socio-political considerations, and the interplay between these. Politically-led agendas, dominant value systems, and resource allocation priorities all have an impact on the type of local services that are provided. Local level service agreements and health care policies, the amount of scope and political will there is to support new initiatives, and the dominant views about how the service should be provided also play a part. An individual clinician's adherence to his or her professional training and the knowledge base that this draws on can have a major influence on how services are delivered. The type of 'expert' role that a clinician decides to take on in his or her work, the extent to which cultural and theoretical diversity is represented in the work setting, and the degree of agency that he or she feels able to exercise in providing culturally appropriate services are other important factors which need to be considered. For many services this may include reducing the language gap experienced by service users who do not speak English by utilising proficient interpreters. Not taking such factors into consideration can lead to discriminatory practices and poor quality health care provision for service users who may need to rely on interpreters (Crawford, 1994; Kaufert et al, 1984; O'Neil et al, 1993).

The need for interpreters

Due to insufficient numbers of bilingual and culturally diverse professional staff groups (Boyle et al, 1993; Marcos, 1979), there continues to be a need for interpreters to bridge the language gap for service users not speaking English (Shackman, 1984; Tribe, 1999). Interpreters play an important role in health care, social welfare, legal, immigration, and commercial work settings (Carr, 1997; Granger, 1996). In Granger and Baker's sample of 64 interpreters about one-third of them worked in mental health settings, with about two-thirds of them working in social welfare and general medical settings. In a few countries such as Canada and Australia there is legislation that requires health care services to be made equally accessible to all sectors of the population, and this extends to a mandate to employ professionally qualified and accredited inter-preters (Carr, 1997). In Britain, Phelan and Parkman (1995) have supported the Audit Commission's recommendation that interpret-ing and communication resources should be made available to all non-English speaking service users. The Health Advisory Commis-sion has advocated that child and adolescent mental health services should give consideration to local population needs when planning services (Health Advisory Service, 1995), so that the needs of the local community are reflected in the types of services that are provided.

The problems associated with misdiagnosing service users due to a lack of linguistic and cultural understanding have been discussed in the mental health literature (e.g. Fernando, 1995; Lau, 1984; Littlewood and Lipsedge, 1989), as has the appropriateness of transferring western psychiatric diagnoses such as Post Traumatic Stress Disorder (PTSD) onto non-western service user populations (Zur, 1996). Such literature has also made a strong case for under-standing mental health problems within a framework utilising the service user's context so that a culturally appropriate understanding is attained (e.g. Lau, 1984; Meyers, 1992; Smail, 1990; Zur, 1994). It has been suggested that emotional connections, identities, and psychological experiences may be dependent on the language being used by a person, and that for bilingual people emotional express-iveness and reporting of psychological difficulties may be manifested very differently depending on whether the first or second language is being used (De Zelueta, 1990, 1995; Marcos et al, 1977; Marcos and Urcuyo, 1979). Also, some psychological states such as those associ-ated with disordered thoughts in a psychotic state are sometimes more apparent in the person's first language (Costillo, 1970). Interpreters therefore have an important task in helping clinicians reach a culturally appropriate and accurate understanding of the service user's psychological difficulties (Cox, 1977). To gain co-operation and treatment compliance clinicians need to understand the illness models held by service users (Crawford, 1994; Kaufert et al, 1985).

In Britain there is marked variation in the quality and delivery of services utilising interpreters. Common practice has been to contract interpreters for discrete pieces of work from a private agency or hospital-based pool. Very few interpreters are employed directly within a particular service. Unfortunately, most health care services are still characterised by insufficient interpreting resources, poor use of trained or untrained interpreters, and the inappropriate use of bilingual staff or family members for interpreting. Corsellis (1997) has argued a case for needing both the organisational support structures, and clinical audit measures at the service level to enhance good work practices utilising interpreters. She suggests the following criteria for effective utilisation of interpreters in mainstream services:

1. Having multidisciplinary teams to ensure communication, service delivery, clinical audit and service development.
2. Ensuring that the right skills have been established in the right place within an organisation.
3. Ensuring that quality services are provided through activities such as

    (a) determining service need and how this matches up with local population demographics (such as the different languages spoken by service users, literacy levels),
    (b) adapting the service to meet the local population need,
    (c) exchanging information and negotiating decisions (by listening to service users, giving adequate information to users),
    (d) providing accessible information about the service to users such as leaflets or videos in different languages, and
    (e) diversifying the service, remembering to accommodate to particular user needs, and monitoring service implementation.

4. Research and development to evaluate the service being provided and support service provision, that is meeting the needs of the local population.

Despite the general acceptance of employing trained interpreters where possible, there still remain models of service provision which are more accepting of non-clinical bilingual staff (e.g. such as ward clerks or secretaries) and volunteers to act as interpreters (Carr, 1997). Calling on bilingual clinical staff such as nurses to interpret, or making use of untrained interpreters, is fraught with many difficulties (Crawford, 1994). Clinical practice utilising untrained volunteers or staff raises both ethical and moral questions, as well as questions about whether service providers are going against the spirit of equal opportunities legislation. In the context of therapy language and meaning are central to the therapeutic work. Mental health work goes beyond the 'simple translation' needed to answer specific social welfare or legal questions. Perhaps it then becomes more important that mental health work is carried out with pro-fessionally trained interpreters.

Training for interpreters and mental health practitioners

The assumption that bilingualism is the main criterion required to work as an interpreter needs challenging (Corsellis, 1997). Accred-ited training for interpreters is gradually on the increase in Britain, although currently there are no legal or professional requirements necessary to secure employment as an interpreter (Roberts, 1997). In the long run certified accreditation should help to empower interpreters in their work by giving them greater professional status (Solomon, 1997). From a postal survey Granger and Baker (Chapter Seven) have noted that whilst many interpreters may hold first degrees (42 per cent) or post-graduate qualifications (28 per cent), usually from their country of origin, very few have undergone any specific training to work as an interpreter (19 per cent); with some having done a short course for interpreters (26 per cent), and many having undertaken no training at all (55 per cent). These results have to be taken with caution as they are based on 64 returned questionnaires from the 300 sent out, and may reflect a skewed sample towards those interpreters who were more fluent in English. Roberts (1997) has pointed out that it is not clear whether formalised training for interpreters should focus on the generic skills required for carrying out translation, or whether there should be some level of specialisation towards the context in which the work would need to be carried out (e.g. legal or health care interpreting).

Suggested topics for courses for interpreters include ethics, counselling theory and therapeutic skills, addressing personal values, roles taken on by interpreters, specialised mental health or medical topics, ways of managing conflict at work, and traditional healing methods (Kaufert and O'Neil, 1995; Roberts, 1997). As most interpreters do not have the financial means or regular work to fund their training, and are likely to have other family and work commitments, there has also been a suggestion that any training offered has to have a degree of flexibility built in to it to enable people to have easier access to it (Kaufert and Koolage, 1984). Kaufert and O'Neil (1995) also identify the need for interpreters to be given support during their training when they experience dilemmas and dissonance arising out of dealing with very different models of health care (e.g. spiritual healing versus counselling strategies, treatment respecting non-violation of body versus invasive medical treatment), and different belief systems (e.g. traditional beliefs about death versus grief model). Interpreters also need support in being able to deal with loyalty issues towards clinicians or service users, managing their anger, and developing strategies to avoid stress or burn out.

Most professional clinical training has limited teaching on race and culture issues. There has been a strong recommendation that clinical psychology training should take more account of race and culture issues (Patel et al, 2000). It has been suggested that minimal training for clinicians or service providers should be aimed at increasing their understanding of the skills needed for translation and interpreting (Penney and Sammons, 1997). However, Corsellis (1997) has suggested that training for clinicians and service providers should include four broad areas:

1. Understanding of the communication process that occurs during communication in a shared language, so that clinicians get a better appreciation about how to communicate more successfully through an interpreter. This would help clinicians develop better ways of using syntax, vocabulary, coding of information, and phrasing.
2. Helping clinicians develop a productive working relationship with interpreters by spending time with them and giving them information which makes their task easier, negotiating decisions, and discussing any intervention with the interpreter before presenting it to the family.

3. Helping clinicians develop ways to adapt the service to meet the needs of the service user.

4. Organisational planning to support the delivery of service across language and culture, as an integral part of the service structure and not a peripheral addition.

A broader training remit for service providers would be aimed at increasing the quality and effectiveness of a service so that equal standards could be applied irrespective of the race or culture of the recipient. The service provider has to ensure that service delivery decisions are based on accurate information, so that he/she is not endangering his/her professional requirements, codes of ethics or good practice, and thereby his/her professional integrity and that of the service. Corsellis (1997) makes the point that race awareness training, which often leaves clinicians with feelings of guilt and anxiety towards working with non-English speaking service users, is no substitute for helping clinicians to become clinically competent in cross-cultural work. Interpreters need to hold positions of greater professional standing in order to have equal parity with clinicians, and one way of ensuring this would be through accredited training for interpreters. However, there should also be an obligation for clinicians to have training in being able to work with interpreters, and maybe to even learn another language in keeping with local population demographics. As well as language training, clinicians need effective cross-cultural training so that they can develop a better contextual understanding of the service user's difficulties, thereby reducing the potential for conflict in the clinical work.

The process of communication and translation

The clinician holds greater power by virtue of speaking English and a technical professional language (Crawford, 1994; Lago and Thompson, 1996). However, power may also be perceived to be with the interpreter by virtue of the interpreter being bilingual and having knowledge of both the clinician's and the service user's culture (Faust and Drickey, 1986). The clinician and the service user are reliant on the interpreter to facilitate communication, and the interpreter is sometimes seen as holding inappropriate power by being able to control the information flow between them. It has also been suggested that the interpreter can empower the service user by facilitating the communication in ways that give the service user a real 'voice' (Harvey, 1984). Viewing the interpreter as an active and important member of the therapeutic interpreter–service user–clinician triad allows for the interpreter's views to be taken into account in a more positive way (Faust and Drickey, 1986; Raval, 1996).

Interpreting requires more than just word for word translation, and advances meaning in the fullest linguistic and cultural sense, so that two people are able to understand each other beyond their words. Interpreters have to elicit information, simplify messages, translate language, introduce information about the service user's cultural context or the service provider's work context, clarify messages, ask for elaboration, introduce choice points into the interaction, explain roles and interaction norms, explain the organisational context, explain the community context, and selectively leave out and translate appropriate information to maximise the understandability of the translation (Kaufert, 1990). The skills required for rendering an accurate translation and conveying information in a meaningful way are not always appreciated by clinicians (Crawford, 1994; Granger, 1996). Strategies such as a change of wording, follow-on questions, letting the service user talk at length, and the use of summary feedback (rather than word for word translation) in order to maintain the flow of conversation are quite helpful for the interpreter. However, clinicians often experience these in negative ways such as feeling that the interpreter is taking control of the session (Raval, 1996). Some of the translation will inevitably contain distortions of meaning depending on how the interpreter has heard the question or comments, and the words that are available for translation (Harvey, 1986). There can be inaccuracies in the translation arising from the omission, addition, or substitution of words (Harvey, 1986; Launer, 1978; Marcos, 1979). Marcos, in evaluating transcripts of psychiatric interviews done with an interpreter, also notes that certain psychiatric questions are difficult for the interpreter to translate accurately without some prior knowledge of psychiatry (e.g. answers to questions relating to thought disorder were normalised by untrained interpreters in their feedback to the psychiatrist). At times the interpreter's attitudes may lead to a distortion in the translation that is given to the clinician.

The temporal processes involved in turn taking, overlap of speech, adjustments needed for translation, the synchrony and flow of conversation are very different when communication has to take place through an interpreter (Roy, 1992). Roy highlights how difficult it is to listen, translate and speak at the same time, and suggests an interpreter using sign language plays an active role in the communication process.

Non-verbal communication varies across cultures and is thought to be shaped by the cultural context that a person grows up in (Lago and Thompson, 1996). Without contextual and cultural understanding and direct linguistic access to the service user, clinicians may find it difficult to understand the non-verbal subtitles and nuances associated with the verbal communication. Rituals may also play a part in communication, and may be misread by clinicians. For example, Freed (1988) in describing her research interviews using an interpreter to talk with Japanese adults who were caring for an elderly relative, felt that having to drink tea before the interviews began was a waste of the limited time available for the research interviews.

Words and metaphors carry different meanings across different cultural contexts. For greater understanding the interpreter and clinician need to have some understanding of the linguistic and cultural world of the service user (Harvey, 1986). Not knowing about the service user's cultural context can lead to misdiagnosis of the service user's problem (Lau, 1984). Having an interpreter can improve the accuracy of a mental health diagnosis and improve the quality of care for the service user (Cox, 1977). Being able to talk in the service user's primary language can encourage positive joining with the service user (De Zelueta, 1990).

The role of the interpreter

There has been much debate in the literature about the role that should be taken on by an interpreter (Kaufert and Koolage, 1984; Kaufert et al, 1985; Roberts, 1997; Wadensjo, 1997, 1998). The roles that have been suggested for interpreters include:

1. Translator (translation is done in a neutral and impartial manner by the interpreter).
2. Cultural broker (interpreter explains and gives cultural and contextual understanding to the clinician or service user).
3. Cultural consultant (interpreter acts as a cultural consultant to the clinician).

4. Advocate for the service user (interpreter represents the service user's interests and speaks on behalf of the user).
5. Intermediary (interpreter mediates on behalf of the clinician or service user).
6. Conciliator (interpreter resolves conflicts which arise between the clinician and the service user).
7. Community advocate (interpreter represents the community concerns at the level of policy making).
8. Link-worker (helps clinicians identify unmet needs of service user, and supportive role with service user to help user make informed choices concerning their health care).
9. Bilingual worker (takes on a more involved therapeutic role in addition to providing translation).

Some authors have suggested that by necessity the interpreter has to take on a variety of roles (Kaufert et al, 1985; Roy, 1992). There is also support for the opposing view held by Marcos (1979) that interpreters should strictly keep to the role of a neutral translator. If an interpreter is viewed as as much a part of the therapeutic system as the clinician and service user then it is difficult to support Marcos's view of the interpreter as being no more than a 'mouth-piece'. From a systemic perspective each member of this triad can be seen as bringing in many influences from their own background to the therapeutic system (Raval, 1996). As bilingual workers, interpreters have much to offer as cultural advisors and cultural brokers, as advocates to the service users, and as advisors and community advocates in relation to health policy making. Inter-preters may need to be explicit in stating this when they are taking on a broader role, but this also needs to be built in to their job descriptions. The work taken on by an interpreter needs to reflect the interpreter's experience, expertise and level of training. This will be difficult to achieve until a proper career structure can be established for interpreters. Conflicts and uncertainties arise when interpreters are not valued or sanctioned by clinicians to take on a broader role, and when interpreters themselves become unsure about taking on a role that goes beyond their job description or level of skill. The advocacy role may be particularly difficult for interpreters when an interpreter has close community or family ties with particular service users (Kaufert and O'Neil, 1995).

Despite the advantages of a more extended and active role for interpreters there remains a dominant theme in the literature about the difficulties that arise in working with interpreters. An extended role for interpreters may be experienced as problematic by clinicians for a number of reasons including:

1. The clinician who is unaccustomed to working with an interpreter or being observed in his/her work may fear being scrutinised (Kline et al, 1980). Holding the view of the interpreter as a neutral conduit and having less direct contact with the service user may lead the clinician to fear a loss of control in the work (Roe and Roe, 1991).
2. Clinicians who fail to acknowledge the skills that an interpreter has in being able to work more independently, and wanting only word for word translation, may feel threatened and unsure about their own role (Freed, 1988)
3. Keeping the interpreter in the role of a neutral conduit may lead to fantasies about what the interpreter is thinking, and the interpreter is more likely to become a transference figure for the clinician's and service user's negative feelings (Harvey, 1984).
4. Conflict may arise when the interpreter is put in the vulnerable position of brokering two sets of irreconcilable viewpoints such as strong biomedical views versus strong cultural perspectives about illness, medical organisational approaches to caring versus traditional views about caring for an ill person, or medical treatment versus traditional healing approaches (Kaufert et al, 1985).
5. Interpreters may find it difficult to work with clinicians who are of a different gender to themselves (Kaufert and Koolage, 1984; Granger, 1996).
6. Clinicians may lack trust in the interpreter's ability to render an accurate translation due to a lack of appreciation of the complexities involved in translation, having to rely on summary information based on the interpreter's conversation with the service user, and not having any direct means to check the content of this conversation (Kaufert and Koolage, 1984).
7. Conflict may arise when the interpreter is taking an advocacy role to enable the service user to make informed choices or give informed consent, particularly when there are polarised views between the clinician and the service user (Kaufert and Koolage, 1984). Informed consent from the service user may be difficult to obtain when there are different cultural norms

about which family member has the authority to give consent, or particular cultural beliefs about protecting the ill family member by withholding information about his or her illness (Kaufert et al, 1996). Clinicians not holding a view that their medical knowledge is culturally and socially constructed, and their lack of cross-cultural training, may add to this conflict (Crawford, 1994).

8. Socio-political influences on service organisation and service delivery, and an unequal power balance in favour of the clinician may make it difficult for the interpreter and service user to have a strong enough voice in influencing the treatment offered to the service user (Kaufert, 1990).

9. Interpreters may find it difficult to work with a service user known to them or provide an accurate translation in this type of situation, as interpreters may want to present their community in a positive light to outside agencies (Freed, 1988).

10. Interpreters may find it difficult to render an accurate translation or may feel uncomfortable when addressing areas such as child abuse or marital discord with the service user (Granger, 1996; Kaufert and Koolage, 1984).

The types of difficulties described above have made it difficult to move towards models of clinical practice allowing the interpreter to play an equal and varied role with clinicians. Perhaps this is going to be more possible when interpreters have accreditation of their training and a better defined professional status.

Issues that arise when conducting therapeutic work with interpreters

The literature contains reports of both positive and negative aspects to the therapeutic work carried out with interpreters. Issues arise for service users, clinicians and interpreters. These have mostly highlighted the difficulties that arise in the work.

Service users have reported the positive impact of interpreters in helping them feel better understood by clinicians and having a sense of the clinician having been helpful to them (Hillier et al, 1994; Kline et al, 1980; Watson, 1984). It is postulated by Kline et al (1980, page 1533) that the service users may have valued the presence of interpreters because they were getting the attention of two people: 'a few drops of water in the desert are infinitely more valued than in a rain forest'. Service users may need time to trust the interpreter and they may have mixed feelings about having to rely on an interpreter to facilitate communication. There may be greater alienation for the service user if the interpreter is seen to be detached and neutral (Roe and Roe, 1991). There may be uncertainties about how the boundaries are defined in the service user's relationship with the interpreter, and a more open relationship with the interpreter and the clinician may be preferable. Negative feelings brought up for service users may be redirected towards the interpreter (Harvey, 1984).

Clinicians have reported both positive and negative experiences of the work with interpreters. Their work is enhanced by the interpreter helping them develop a better cultural understanding about the service user, helping them gain greater communication and engagement with the service user, and helping them obtain accurate information about the service user (Raval, 1996). In contrast, certain taboo topics such as abuse, and making psychiatric diagnoses are experienced as being more difficult in the presence of an interpreter. Clinicians may also report greater detachment from the service user, feel less powerful in relation to the work, and feel less effective in their work (Kline et al, 1980; Raval, 1996).

Clinicians have often viewed the interpreter as an added complication to their work (Faust and Drickey, 1986). Clinicians often feel frustrated because the work takes more time (Crawford, 1994; Freed, 1988; Raval, 1996). Kline et al (1980) have reported on the experience of junior psychiatrists who saw some Spanish-speaking service users with an interpreter and other Spanish-speaking service users without an interpreter. The junior psychiatrists misread the extent to which service users had felt understood and helped when seen with an interpreter. Kline et al suggest possible explanations for why the junior psychiatrists felt more pessimistic about those service users seen with an interpreter: (a) the psychiatrists preferred direct one-to-one contact with service users and felt better able to work with the transference; (b) they were worried about maintaining the confidentiality for the service user, and they felt scrutinised by the interpreter thus doubting their abilities even more as they were still in training; and (c) the psychiatrists were holding racist attitudes. These authors conclude that the psychiatrists' misjudgement arose not out of 'crude anti-Hispanic prejudice but from difficulties we all experience in bridging cultural and linguistic barriers' (Kline et al, 1980, page 1533).

The major issues for interpreters have touched on themes related to not being appreciated in the work they do, and not having professional recognition (Crawford, 1994; Granger, 1996; Kaufert and Koolage, 1984; Tribe, 1999). Interpreters report having little power in relation to clinicians, having an unclear professional status, a lack of recognition of the work they do, and poor support structures in the work setting. Interpreters value having greater autonomy in their work. There is greater resentment amongst professional staff such as nurses who are asked to interpret. Interpreters find it difficult to manage the emotional impact of their work particularly when they are not given supervisory or peer group support. Managing triangulated relationships, adjusting to the variability of different clinicians and their working styles, developing a sense of their own professional identity, and having to deal with the cultural insensitivity of clinicians is difficult for interpreters. Sometimes, interpreters find themselves alienated from their community due to their bilingualism, where being able to speak English as a second language is seen as representing social mobility or selling out to the dominant culture (Crawford, 1994).

Granger and Baker (Chapter Seven) have found that more experienced interpreters are likely to see the need for training for themselves as well as for other professionals, and the need to be given sufficient information by clinicians to enable them to work more effectively. Interpreters in Granger and Baker's study reported that interpreting was a skilled task requiring them to have flexibility, adaptability, interpersonal skills, tact, sensitivity, intuition, empathy, objectivity, diplomacy, intelligence, patience, tolerance, negotiating skills, ability to build up trust, having to adjust to the clinician's lack of training in being able to work with them, ability to convey emotional and linguistic information, and ability to draw on knowledge held by the clinician and the service user. The problems encountered by interpreters included clinicians not being given sufficient information about the service user, not being allocated enough pre- and post-session time to discuss the work, a lack of continuity and trust when they are only required for one-off appointments, and unclear expectations from the clinician about each other's roles. Interpreters may find it harder to remain objective when they know that they are the only link that the service user has with the outside world. Practical factors like poor pay, travelling across different service settings, lack of regular and predictable work, and delays in getting paid or reimbursed for expenses make their job physically and emotionally demanding. Whilst 86 per cent of Granger and Baker's sample were satisfied with their job as an interpreter, 64 per cent were willing to change their job, and 50 per cent of them reported feeling valued by other professionals.

Ethical considerations for the work of interpreters

Solomon (1997, p. 88) suggests that a definition of ethics as 'morally sensitive persons in particular situations' helps with overriding the dogma of ethical guidelines, and makes them more workable when bridging the cultural and linguistic gap. He suggests that ethical guidelines for interpreters need to be more responsive. Ethical guidelines have been developed for interpreters and the broad areas covered in these mainly North American guidelines (Kaufert and Putsch, 1997; Roe and Roe, 1991; Solomon, 1997) include:

1. Confidentiality: interpreters have to ensure confidentiality for the service user.
2. Accuracy: interpreters have to render the translation faithfully, conveying the content and the spirit of the speaker using language most readily understood by the person being served.
3. Completeness: interpreters must interpret everything that is said by all people in the interaction, but should inform health professionals if the content might be perceived as offensive, intrusive or harmful to the dignity and well-being of the service user.
4. Appropriateness of work undertaken: interpreters should accept assignments using discretion with regards to skills, setting, and the service user involved. Interpreters should disclose any real or perceived conflict that would affect their objectivity in the delivery of the service.
5. Convey cultural frameworks: when appropriate interpreters should explain cultural differences to health providers and service users.
6. Non-judgmental attitude: an interpreter's function is to facilitate communication. Just as interpreters should not omit anything being said, they should also not add their own personal opinions, advice or judgement.
7. Self-determination for service user: the service user may ask the interpreter for his or her opinion. The interpreter should not

influence the opinion of the service user or their family by telling them what action to take.

8. Attitude towards service user: the interpreter should strive to develop a relationship of trust and respect at all times with the service user by adopting a caring, attentive, and impartial attitude towards the service user and their questions, concerns, and needs.

9. Compensation: the fee or the salary paid by the agency is the only compensation that the interpreter should accept. Interpreters should not accept additional money, considerations or favours for services.

Solomon (1997) has welcomed ethical guidelines for interpreters but has criticised the value placed on individual self-determination, as there are cultural differences in the extent to which the individual concerns are balanced against the principles of respect, dignity, and humanity of individuals in the context of the social, physical, cultural, and psychological interconnections that shape individual lives. In many cultures less emphasis is placed on self-determination and needing to know the 'truth' about one's illness. Also, the view that the interpreter holds a neutral position has been questioned with regards to the multiple roles that an interpreter can take on, which at times would necessitate the interpreter to have clear views about what is in the best interests of the service user.

Kaufert and Putsch (1997) have criticised the guidelines for failing to take a broader cultural perspective and instead staying very much within a western cultural framework. They argue that such guidelines perpetuate the view of an interpreter as a peripheral ancillary staff member who is not neutral, and who needs constant checking to make sure that he or she is not censoring information. They argue that in practice interpreters cannot be neutral as they have to render meaning to the explanatory models held by clinicians and service users, based on their own understanding. Instead ethical guidelines should encourage interpreters to be more transparent in their work, leaving room for open discussion by all the parties concerned. Kaufert and Putsch also note that given the complexities involved in the process of interpreting, the notion of the interpreter as a neutral translator is unrealistic in actual clinical practice.

Summary

In a mental health care context where cultural and language diversity is poorly represented amongst professional staff groups, interpreters continue to provide an important service to bridge the resulting language gap for non-English speaking service users. Therapeutic work carried out with an interpreter can lead to many benefits for both clinicians and service users, but is also fraught with difficulties. Many of these difficulties seem to arise due to inadequate training opportunities for interpreters and clinicians, and no mandatory requirement for such training. They may also arise when the role being taken on in the work by the interpreter is not properly negotiated by the clinician. There remains a tension between employing an interpreter to work exclusively as a translator and in allowing an interpreter to develop a broader remit as a bilingual worker. Services making use of interpreters need to develop greater respect for the work that they do, and move towards models of in-house employment of interpreters. Formalised training would help towards the professionalisation of interpreters. Accredited training courses and ethical guidelines are beginning to be developed for interpreters working in Britain.

The literature in this area of work is restricted and largely limited to descriptive reports about the difficulties that arise in the clinical work when done with the help of an interpreter. There is a need for research in this area of work, and a need to develop a theoretical grounding from which to inform the clinical practice with interpreters.

References

Aitken, G. (1998) 'Reflections on working with and across difference: race and personal differences in clinical psychology encounters'. *Clinical Psychology Forum*, 128: 11–17.

Boyle, M., Baker, M., Bennett, E. and Charman, T. (1993) 'Selection for clinical psychology training courses; a comparison of applicants from ethnic minority and majority groups to the University of East London'. *Clinical Psychology Forum*, 56: 9–13.

Carr, S. E. (1997) 'A three-tiered health care interpreter system'. In S. E. Carr, R. Roberts, A. Dufour and D. Steyn (eds), *The Critical Link: Interpreters in the Community*. Philadelphia: John Benjamins Publishing Company, pp. 271–276.

Corsellis, A. (1997) 'Training needs of public personnel working with interpreters'. In S. E. Carr, R. Roberts, A. Dufour and D. Steyn (eds), *The Critical Link: Interpreters in the Community*. Philadelphia: John Benjamins Publishing Company, pp. 77–89.

Costillo, J. (1970) 'The influence of language upon symptomatology in foreign-born patients'. *American Journal of Psychiatry*, 127: 242–244.

Cox, J. (1977) 'Aspects of transcultural psychiatry'. *British Journal of Psychiatry*, 130: 211–221.

Crawford, A. (1994) 'Black patients/white doctors: stories lost in translation'. Paper presented at National Language Project, 1st World Congress of African Linguistics, Kwaluseni, Swaziland.

De Zelueta, F. (1990) 'Bilingualism and family therapy'. *Journal of Family Therapy*, 12: 255–265.

De Zelueta, F. (1995) 'Bilingualism, culture and identity'. *Group Analysis*, 28: 179–190.

Drennan, G. (1999) 'Psychiatry, post-apartheid integration and the neglected role of language in South African institutional contexts'. *British Journal of Psychiatry*, 36: 5–22.

Faust, S. and Drickey, R. (1986) 'Working with interpreters'. *Journal of Family Practice*, 22: 131–138.

Fernando, S. (1995) *Mental Health in a Multi-Ethnic Society*. London: Routledge.

Freed, A. (1988) 'Interviewing through an interpreter'. *Social Work*, July/August 1988: 315–319.

Goodman, R. and Scott, S. (1997) *Child Psychiatry*. London: Blackwell Science.

Granger, E. (1996) 'A psychological investigation into the role and work experience of the interpreter'. Unpublished thesis submitted for Doctoral Degree in Clinical Psychology, University of East London.

Harvey, M. (1984) 'Family therapy with deaf persons: the systemic utilisation of an interpreter'. *Family Process*, 23: 205–213.

Harvey, M. A. (1986) 'The magnifying mirror: family therapy for deaf persons'. *Family Systems Medicine*, 4: 408–420.

Health Advisory Service (1995) *Child and Adolescent Mental Health Services: Together We Stand (Commissioning, role, and management of child and adolescent mental health services)*. London: HMSO.

Herbert, M. (1991) *Clinical Child Psychology*. Chichester: John Wiley and Sons.

Hillier S., Huq, A., Loshak, R., Marks, F. and Rahman, S. (1994) 'An evaluation of child psychiatric services for Bangladeshi parents'. *Journal of Mental Health*, 3: 332–337.

Kaufert, J. M. (1990) 'Sociological and anthropological perspectives on the impact of interpreters on clinician/client communication'. *Santé Culture Health*, VII (2–3): 209–235.

Kaufert, J. M. and Koolage, W. W. (1984) 'Role conflict among cultural brokers: the experience of native Canadian medical interpreters'. *Social Science Medicine*, 18: 283–286.

Kaufert, J. M. and O'Neil, J. D. (1995) 'Cultural mediation of dying and grieving among native Canadian patients in urban hospitals'. In L. A. DeSpelder and A. L. Strickland (eds), *The Path Ahead: Readings in Death and Dying*. Mountain View, CA: Mayfield Publishing Company.

Kaufert, J. M. and Putsch, R. W. (1997) 'Communication through interpreters in healthcare: ethical dilemmas arising from differences in class, culture, language, and power'. *The Journal of Clinical Ethics*, 8: 71–87.

Kaufert, J. M., O'Neil, J. D. and Koolage, W. W. (1985) 'Culture brokerage and advocacy in urban hospitals: the impact of native language interpreters'. *Santé Culture Health*, VII(2–3): 3–9.

Kaufert, J. M., Koolage, W. W., Kaufert, P. L. and O'Neil, J. D. (1984) 'The use of "trouble case" examples in teaching the impact of sociocultural and political factors in clinical communication'. *Medical Anthropology*, 8: 36–45.

Kaufert, J., Lavallee, M., Koolage, W. and O'Neil, J. (1996) 'Culture and informed consent: the role of Aboriginal interpreters in patient advocacy in urban hospitals'. *Issues In The North*, 1: 89–92.

Kline, F., Acosta, F., Austin, W. and Johnson, R. G. (1980) 'The misunderstood Spanish-speaking patient'. *American Journal of Psychiatry*, 137: 1530–1533.

Lago, C. and Thompson, J. (1996) *Race, Culture and Counselling*. Buckingham: Open University Press.

Lau, A. (1984) 'Transcultural issues in family therapy'. *Journal of Family Therapy*, 6: 91–112.

Launer, J. (1978) 'Taking medical histories through interpreters: practice in a Nigerian outpatient department'. *British Medical Journal*, 2: 934–935.

Littlewood, R. and Lipsedge, M. (1989) *Aliens and Alienists: Ethnic Minorities and Psychiatry*. London: Unwin Hyman Ltd.

Marcos, L. (1979) 'Effects of interpreters on the psychopathology in non-English-speaking patients'. *American Journal of Psychiatry*, 136: 171–174.

Marcos, L. R. and Urcuyo, L. (1979) 'Dynamic psychotherapy with bilingual patients'. *American Journal of Psychotherapy*, XXXIII: 331–338.

Marcos, L. R., Eisma, J. E. and Guimon, J. (1977) 'Bilingualism and sense of self'. *The American Journal of Psychoanalysis*, 37: 285–290.

Meyers, C. (1992) 'Hmong children and their families: consideration of cultural influences in assessment'. *The American Journal of Occupational Therapy*, 46: 737–744.

O'Neil, J. D., Kaufert, J. M., Kaufert, P. L. and Koolage, W. W. (1993)

'Political considerations in health-related participatory research in northern Canada'. In N. Dyck and J. B. Waldram (eds), *Anthropology, Public Policy, and Native Peoples in Canada*. Montreal: McGill Queens University Press, pp. 216–232.

Patel, N., Bennett, E., Dennis, M., Dosanjh, N., Mahtani, A., Miller A. and Nairdshaw, Z. (2000) *Clinical Psychology 'Race' and Culture: A Training Manual*. Leicester: British Psychological Society Books.

Penney, C. and Sammons, S. (1997) 'Training the community interpreter: the Nunavut Arctic College experience'. In S. E. Carr, R. Roberts, A. Dufour and D. Steyn (eds), *The Critical Link: Interpreters in the Community*. Philadelphia: John Benjamins Publishing Company, pp. 65–76.

Phelan, M. and Parkman, S. (1995) 'Working with an interpreter'. *British Medical Journal*, 311: 555–557.

Raval, H. (1996) 'A systemic perspective on working with interpreters'. *Clinical Child Psychology and Psychiatry*, 1: 29–43.

Ridley, R. R. (1995) *Overcoming Unintentional Racism in Counselling and Therapy*. Thousand Oaks, CA: Sage Publications.

Roberts, R. P. (1997) 'Community interpreting today and tomorrow'. In S. E. Carr, R. Roberts, A. Dufour and D. Steyn (eds), *The Critical Link: Interpreters in the Community*. Philadelphia: John Benjamins Publishing Company, pp. 7–26.

Roe, D. and Roe, C. (1991) 'The third party: using interpreters for the deaf in counselling situations'. *Journal of Mental Health Counselling*, 13: 91–105.

Roy, C. B. (1992) 'A socio-linguistic analysis of the interpreter's role in simultaneous talk in a face-to-face interpreted dialogue'. *Sign Language Studies*, 5: 21–61.

Rutter, M. and Hersov, L. (1985) *Child Adolescent Psychiatry*. London: Blackwell.

Shackman, J. (1984) *The Right to be Understood. A Handbook on Working with, Employing and Training Community Interpreters*. Cambridge: National Extension College.

Smail, D. (1990) 'Design for a post-behaviourist clinical psychology'. *Clinical Psychology Forum*, 22: 2–10.

Solomon, M. Z. (1997) 'From what's neutral to what's meaningful: reflections on a study of medical interpreters'. *The Journal of Clinical Ethics*, 8: 88–93.

Tribe, R. (1999) 'Bridging the gap or damming the flow? Using interpreters/bicultural workers when working with refugee clients, many of whom have been tortured'. *British Journal of Medical Psychology*, 72: 567–576.

Wadensjo, C. (1997) 'Recycled information as a questioning strategy: pitfalls in interpreter-mediated talk'. In S. E. Carr, R. Roberts, A.

Dufour and D. Steyn (eds), *The Critical Link: Interpreters in the Community*. Philadelphia: John Benjamins Publishing Company.

Wadensjo, C. (1998) *Interpreting As Interaction*. New York: Longman.

Watson, E. (1984) 'Health of infants and use of health services by mothers of different ethnic groups in East London'. *Community Medicine*, 6: 127–135.

Wetherell, M. and Potter, J. (1992) *Mapping The Language of Racism: Discourse and the Legitimation of Exploitation*. Hemel Hempstead: Harvester Wheatsheaf.

Zur, J. (1994) 'The psychological impact of impunity'. *Anthropology Today*, 10: 12–17.

Zur, J. (1996) 'From PTSD to voices in context: from an "experience-far" to an "experience-near" understanding of responses to war and atrocity across cultures'. *International Journal of Social Psychiatry*, 42: 305–317.

Chapter 2

Interpreters in medical consultations

Annie Cushing

Interpreters

In this chapter the term interpreter refers to bilingual interpreters trained to work with health professionals and service users to enable each side to understand the other, with the aim of arriving at a shared understanding of the problem and possible solutions. Confusion can arise over the different terms of translator, interpreter and advocate, which are sometimes used interchangeably. Translation involves converting words of one language to another. In the field of court interpretation programmes, it is essential not to violate the rule of accurate translation. However, in the medical context the aim is to achieve mutual understanding and is not normally adversarial. In this situation, whilst it is important that the meaning is not distorted and that the interpreter is not adding or omitting information, the interpreter will be choosing words and explanations to convey accurately the meaning of concepts. She[1] will need to be familiar with medical terminology and ask for clarification when she does not understand. Advocacy involves empowerment in enabling service users to get information and to access services that they need. Advocates' roles are not only to interpret, but to educate health workers about the culture and health problems of service users, assist service users in understanding procedures and services, provide appropriate health education, and enable service users to understand options open to them. In both primary care and hospital settings advocates may undertake

---

[1] Throughout this chapter, the interpreter is referred to as 'she' and the service user as 'he'.

screening interviews and give some health advice, as well as sit in on consultations.

Interpreters' training will have included ethical aspects of the role. Central to this is strict confidentiality, faithful interpretation, impartiality and respect for service users and providers with commitment to service user self-determination, and avoidance of inappropriate expression of personal opinion or advice (Hardt, 1995).

The term 'interpreter' will be used in this chapter but it should already be evident that the roles and boundaries of the task may vary, and that there is considerable potential for helping service users and health professionals as well as the possibility of problems arising when the health professional is uncertain about what role the interpreter is taking.

The consultation

Any consultation is a social interaction in which roles are assumed by each side, where status and power are implicit if not explicit. This interaction always brings together two cultures: that of the service user with a set of lay beliefs, language, experiences and expectations, and that of the health professional with a biomedical knowledge and specialised language for interpreting and managing the illness process. The consultation involves the meeting of these two explanatory models. Superimpose on this social class, education, gender, religious, language, race and ethnic differences between service user and helper and the process can be seen to be complex (see Figure 2.1).

Tuckett et al (1985) talk about shared meaning as a goal for a consultation. Both sides coming from different perspectives are able to understand each other and develop a shared way of discussing the same problem. In many cases it should be possible to attain mutual agreement and satisfaction with decisions reached, although in some instances service users' and health professionals' cultural values are irreconcilable (Kaufert and Putsch, 1997).

Tuckett showed, however, that in 'same language' consultations service users' views were rarely sought by doctors, that service users mostly did not disclose their thoughts, or if they did, the doctors often interrupted or dismissed this information. Although in the majority of cases doctors did provide explanations and information, they rarely checked whether service users had

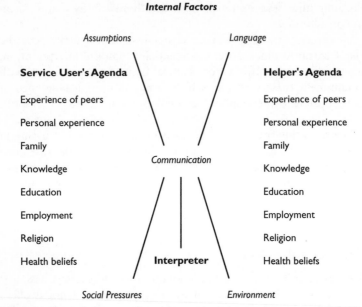

Figure 2.1   Factors influencing communication

understood. More recent research on informed consent supports these findings (Levinson et al, 1997).

Hence we can already see there may be problems in doctors understanding service users and in service users understanding doctors even before ethnic background and language barriers are considered.

Power, control and the doctor–service user relationship

Why do doctors not explore the service users' agenda more often? They may be underestimating the importance of the service users' perspective and psychosocial aspects of health problems (Engel, 1977). Alternatively, doctors' behaviour could be a function of attempts, conscious or otherwise, to maintain authority in the relationship and increase their power to reassure (Maguire, 1984). Time is cited as a constraining factor in consultations and doctors will inevitably work on assumptions about service users, which may or may not be correct. Waitzkin (1985) found that the belief sometimes held by health professionals, that working class service users want less information about their illnesses, was based on people's hesitancy in asking questions rather than an actual disinterest in having information.

Why do service users not offer their views or ask questions more often? The status given to health professionals means people may accept what they say unquestioningly, or if they disagree they do so silently. The power imbalance in the doctor–service user situation does not enable the service user to feel free to express feelings and ideas (Davis and Fallowfield, 1990). To change this doctors would have to provide service users with information that demystifies the situation, request feedback from the service user, and actively welcome service users' questions (Roter, 1979).

Sociological research identifies a number of models of the doctor–service user relationship. The expert model describes the relationship where the doctor, who has medical diagnostic and treatment expertise, decides what is best, prescribes treatment, and expects the service user to follow advice without any reference to the service user's perspective (Cunningham and Davis, 1985; Szasz and Hollander, 1956). Service user expectations of the omnipotent doctor may have matched and reinforced this model (Boreham and Gibson, 1978).

In contrast the partnership approach, also termed the mutual participation model, acknowledges the service user as expert in their own lives, values the service user's autonomy and self-determination, and encourages the person to take part in problem definition and treatment decisions (Tuckett et al, 1985). The interviewing style which matches this is service user centred. The doctor tries to understand not only the biomedical process but also the meaning and experience of the illness for the service user (McWhinney, 1989). In western health care the cultural norm is away from the paternalistic style of consultation to one based on service user autonomy and self-determination. Fundamental to this approach and enshrined in the duties of a doctor is truth-telling, maintaining service user confidentiality and informed consent (Doyal, 1996; General Medical Council, 1998).

When a service user and health professional meet confusion occurs if there are differences in expectations and uncertainties about how each party behaves in the consultation, or if each side expects a different outcome (Bochner, 1982). Hence even when the language and societal culture of the service user and doctor are similar, there is still a gap of lay and medical culture and power to be bridged. This is even more the case when the service user speaks a different language and comes from an ethnic group with potentially dissimilar explanatory models, life experiences, cultural values, expectations, and group and family relationships to the dominant culture.

The advantages of using trained interpreters over using family members, friends or bilingual hospital staff do not therefore just relate to confidentiality and accuracy of reporting. The trained medical interpreter spans the two cultures with one foot in the service user's culture and the other in the health professional's medical culture. Hence they are able to translate, act as culture broker in explaining and helping both sides to understand each other, and act as the service user's advocate.

Effective communication in the consultation

Bird and Cohen-Cole (1990) describe the consultation as having three functions: building a collaborative relationship; obtaining a clear picture of the problem; and explaining the doctor's diagnosis and proposed management with the aim of negotiating a plan which both sides can feel committed to. Behaviours which help fulfil these functions are identified in Table 2.1. An interpreter has to fulfil these three functions.

Challenges and issues in communication between service users and health professionals, which interpreters help with, will be discussed in the following areas:

- *Language and translation* (e.g. lack of words for some conditions, culturally sanctioned forms of verbal and non-verbal expressions)
- *Concepts of health and illness* (connection between physical and psychological symptoms, social and cultural factors in illness causation and experience)
- *Communication styles* (verbal and non-verbal communication and the social meaning that they convey)

Table 2.1   Three functions in a consultation – behaviours that help

1. Building a relationship – to promote positive partnership	2. Accurate and comprehensive information gathering – to define the problems in the context of the service user's life	3. Education and management – to achieve shared understanding and agreed treatment plan
Environment – privacy, seating Names Orientation – roles, purpose of meeting, confidentiality Empathy Respect Support and encouragement Appropriate reassurance Non-judgmental – open mindedness, accept the person even if you don't approve of the behaviour	Simple questions Open questions Unbiased questions Attentive listening Clarification Summarising Organising interview – redirecting and signposting	Explore service user's beliefs, feelings, expectations Explain your own views Invite questions Explore service user's reaction to this Clarify common ground Negotiate agreed plan Ask for feedback – ask service user to repeat and affirm the plan

- *The doctor–service user relationship* (paternalism to autonomy; status, power and deference; trust and confidentiality; fear of disapproval; gender)
- *Taboo areas* which may be difficult to talk about (bodily parts and functions, mental illness, terminal illness).

Language and translation

A trained medical interpreter is essential to get accurate exchange of information (Hornberger et al, 1997). Psychological or psycho-social problems are detected more often in a consultation with an interpreter present (Blochliger et al, 1997). Interpreting can be done using simultaneous interpretation or more usually consecutive interpretation. More utterances on the part of the doctor and service user with fewer misunderstandings have been reported with simultaneous interpretations. However, whilst service users and clinicians preferred this method, bilingual interpreters preferred the consecutive method (Hornberger et al, 1996). Simultaneous translation is difficult and requires intensive training with attention to linguistics and memory.

Marcos (1979) points to the danger of 'normalisation', which can occur in the consecutive method of interpretation and states that mental health consultations can particularly benefit from simultaneous interpretations where the service users' thoughts are disorganised. If interpreters are unaware of the importance of this information for diagnosis they may leave it out.

DOCTOR: What is the problem?

INTERPRETER: What is the problem?

SERVICE USER: The room is spinning round me, I feel sick and I have a pain in my stomach. There are spirits who are making me ill for the bad deed I did to my neighbour.

INTERPRETER: He feels dizzy and sick and has pain in his stomach.

In this interaction a literal translation would raise for the doctor a possibility of a psychiatric problem. The interpreter may censor the last part because she knows that people from this culture believe physical illness to be caused by misdeeds. If the health professional is unaware of the cultural variation in how symptoms are revealed then a literal translation may be misinterpreted.

Whilst it is important that meaning is not distorted by the interpreter, Kaufert and Koolage (1984) argue that objective neutrality in the interpretation may actually reduce the value of interpreters to service users and doctors. Interpreters are needed to establish rapport and find culturally appropriate analogies for complex biomedical terminology used in consultations.

Another problem which has been identified is the situation where the words used are not equivalent in meaning:

DOCTOR: What has your mood been like recently?

INTERPRETER: How have you been feeling recently?

SERVICE USER: Since I have been taking the medicine the pain has gone and my stomach feels fine.

INTERPRETER: She feels fine. Her stomach is better since taking the medicine.

In this instance the doctor must ensure the interpreter understands the importance of the concept of mood and is able to find ways of conveying this.

Codes of practice for interpreters emphasise accuracy, neutrality, achieving a balance between speakers, and intervening personally only in three types of situations (Language Line, 1998):

- to ask for clarification of concept, jargon, vocabulary or services and institutions which do not translate well
- to request adjustment of delivery e.g. pace and volume
- alerting the service provider to a situation where the user has not understood.

Medical interpreters will inevitably develop medical knowledge as a result of frequent translation. As one interpreter said:

> Sometimes I know the service user is concerned about something, and I could answer it but I think it is important for the doctor to know and to answer it herself. I will therefore tell the doctor that the service user is worried about this particular problem so that she can explain through me.

In this way the interpreter is not just translating at the point of interaction but bringing to the doctor's attention questions which she knows the service user is concerned about or has not understood.

Case example

A doctor wanted to explain to a pregnant woman of 36 weeks' gestation with raised blood pressure and $^{+++}$ *protein in her urine that she needed admission to hospital.*

DOCTOR: *Your blood pressure is high. You need to come into hospital so we can check on you for the safety of your baby.*

INTERPRETER: *Your blood pressure is high. You need to come into hospital so we can check on you for the safety of your baby.*

WOMAN: *No, I don't want to come into hospital. I feel very well, my baby is moving and I am better at home. I cannot eat well in hospital and I cannot be with my family. They will look after me and I can rest at home.*

INTERPRETER: *She does not want to come in because she feels well and thinks her baby is fine. She wants to be with her family and is worried about the food in hospital.*

DOCTOR: *It is very important for the health of your baby that we check your blood pressure.*

INTERPRETER: *Your blood pressure is high and your urine shows that this could be causing a strain on your kidneys. This may stop your baby growing and could be dangerous for your baby. Your blood pressure may settle down fine but in hospital the doctors can check it often and if there is still a problem they can decide what to do. Your family can visit and we can discuss your food needs with you.*

SERVICE USER: *Alright.*

INTERPRETER: *She says yes.*

Such lengthy exchanges sometimes worry doctors who wonder what is being said. However, here the interpreter is drawing upon her experience of having worked in this clinic for some time, ensuring the woman understands the importance whilst not wanting to alarm her, and trying to address her concerns. Kaufert and Koolage (1984) found that often interpreters needed to move beyond the direct translation of the concept to explain the function of an organ or describe a procedure in lay language.

Concepts of health and illness

Socio-cultural factors of importance include the meaning of health in a community, the meaning of mental health, medical belief system, beliefs about death and dying, attitudes about pregnancy, childbirth, childcare, and sexual behaviour amongst others. An interpreter who comes from the same culture or background as the service user may be able to help in explaining cultural beliefs and expectations.

Beliefs about illness and its causation may range from bad luck, karma and punishment for misdeeds, the will of another person, God's will, biomedical and scientific explanations, lifestyle and environment (Quereshi, 1988). Within the same cultural group beliefs and behaviour can vary enormously and individuals do not always share the same concepts so it is important to keep an open mind.

It is sometimes said that there is no concept of depression in some cultures and no language to convey this. Distress is experienced as physical symptoms and people may expect a physical treatment of their problem even though doctors suspect psychological causes.

Table 2.2   Relevant issues for mental health

What is the traditional or local name (if any)?
What is its western medical name (if any)?
What are its symptoms? Its cause(s)?
What type of person(s) does the mental illness usually affect?
Can it be prevented, and if so, how?
How is it diagnosed? Treated? Cured?
What types of practitioners or other individuals are best able to prevent,
   diagnose, and/or treat the mental illness
What methods are generally used by each?
What are the views towards counselling?
What are the typical attitudes to this mental illness and the person who has it?
Are there taboos or other beliefs connected with mental illness?
What are the typical community attitudes towards mental illness?
Is mental illness caused or influenced by cultural readjustment?
How are the mentally ill cared for by their families and others in the
   community?
What attitudes do members hold towards receiving help for mental or
   emotional problems?
Are certain types of treatment more acceptable and more likely to be
   successful?

Source: Randall-David (1989)

Translation of medical conditions may have no meaning and convey nothing of the characteristics or implications of these labels (Jackson et al, 1997). On the other hand people do find many ways to communicate but professionals are not always aware of what these are. Fuller and Toon (1988) refers to the syndrome of 'total body pain' as a symptom of psychological distress, which is particularly common in some cultural groups.

Issues of particular relevance for the mental health consultation are listed in Table 2.2 (Randall-David, 1989). Mental illness carries stigma in any culture. However, some countries and cultures label and recognise it more than others. In cultures where greater regard is placed on genetic causes of mental illness, such a diagnosis can have enormous social implications for marriage and a diagnosis of mental illness may well be resisted. Talking with interpreters may provide health workers with information which then has a bearing on the consultation.

Not infrequently loss of status, fear of being seen as a failure, and shame accompany seeking help for mental health problems. There may be considerable differences in talking about one's family problems with a stranger; some groups being very expressive, whilst others are more closed. These factors will influence the process of the consultation. Attention to demonstrating respect, acknowledging difficulty, reassurance, and indicating the reason for a particular line of questioning is needed.

It is evident from this that the interpreter has an important role in being able to mediate between the biomedical model of the doctor and the cultural belief system, and its expression, of the service user.

Communication styles

How people express symptoms and the way health professionals interpret this in their clinical reasoning is a subject of interest in sociological research (Todd and Fisher, 1993). A recent study investigated why South Asian people in the UK experience greater delays than Europeans in obtaining appropriate specialist management for heart disease (Chaturvedi et al, 1997). There were no differences in perceived implications of symptoms between Europeans and South Asian people and indeed the latter were more likely to want to seek care in the case of such symptoms. The authors concluded that service-related explanations must be explored, including the process of the consultation. They stated that delays were unlikely to be due to overt racism, given that many service users consult a general practitioner from their own ethnic group, but hypothesised that subtle cultural differences in expressing symptoms and the difficulty with which these symptoms are interpreted and acted upon by Western-trained doctors might be more likely to cause delay. Clearly further research is needed, but this study does highlight the potential importance of communication style in cross-cultural communication.

Fuller and Toon (1988) point out how differences in levels of stoicism and emotional expression occur between cultural groups and also the dangers of stereotyping and assumptions which these can engender. A clinician from a stoical society may fail to take seriously the complaint of a service user from a more emotional culture.

Non-verbal communication

In any conversation much information is conveyed by non-verbal means. Establishing rapport helps information exchange and can be therapeutic in itself (Novack, 1995). It helps if social behaviour such as distance and body space, handshaking, body movements, eye contact, forms of address and titles which convey respect and politeness or hostility and disrespect can be anticipated. Social conventions vary. Linguistic conventions such as 'please' and 'thank you' that are extremely important in some cultures do not exist in other groups. Frequent use of such terms may be interpreted as superficial and insincere. Absence of such terms may be experienced by health providers as rudeness.

To avoid confrontation, disrespect, disagreement, frustration or even anger, some cultures are indirect, indifferent, silent or may smile reluctantly. Smiling or laughing may mask other emotions or avoid conflict. Deference to others may be common. Personal feelings may not be disclosed when emotional expressions are seen as a sign of immaturity and stoicism is valued. In contrast to this other cultures encourage emotional expression. We gain information from body language such as facial expression, gestures, posture, position, touch and eye contact. Aspects of speech such as tone of voice, stress and emphasis, pauses and pace of speech (collectively called prosody) also provide information. Silence, for example, may be interpreted as someone lost in feelings, or if it follows a question may be taken as a sign that they have not understood. However, in some cultures it is a sign of respect to wait after a question before answering and not that the person is confused or has failed to understand (Brislin and Yoshida, 1994). Long periods of silence are comfortable with some groups, whilst in others people speak before someone has finished talking. All of this points to the need for checking with the service user what he has understood and how he is feeling.

In the field of mental health the service user's demeanour and affect are important aspects in diagnosis. The health provider may not be able to 'read' the service user and the interpreter may be able to give them a more accurate interpretation of what this non-verbal behaviour indicates. An important principle, however, is for the health provider not to discuss the service user with the interpreter during the consultation without involving the service user.

The doctor–service user relationship

The expectations of a service user from a different culture may be different from someone of the same culture as the health provider. The interpreter has an advocacy role in this situation. They may ask questions on behalf of the service user. Sometimes these are questions which the service user has asked at a pre-consultation meeting and are perhaps questions which the interpreter herself could answer, but it is more appropriate that the health professional hears and answers them within the consultation.

Some service users want health professionals to take control, give explicit directions on how to solve problems, and bring immediate relief from their symptoms. The health professional adopting a partnership approach and biopsychosocial model of health care may be seen as uncertain, and not knowing what is wrong or what should be done. Others want just such an approach. Whilst anecdotes abound there has been no systematic research on the expectations of different cultural groups.

Some research has shown that service users from ethnic minority groups get shorter consultations (Tuckett et al, 1985) and are more likely to get a prescription (Gill et al, 1995). The explanation may be complex but it does indicate that something different is happening in these consultations. Whether it is the health professional, service user, or the general uncertainty of the interaction driving this behaviour is not clear.

Taboo areas

It is in the area of culture-bound values, where those of the health professionals and service users differ, that interpreters have been found to experience considerable role conflict (Kaufert and Koolage, 1984). In situations of serious and terminal illness medical interpreters can find themselves caught between strongly-held core cultural values and ethical principles of the community and health profession.

Kaufert and Koolage point out that Western notions of the sovereignty of the individual person and individual life can come into direct conflict with alternative values, namely where the good or primacy of the community takes precedence over individual autonomy. Strong cultural prohibitions on telling service users bad news have been described (Carrese and Rhodes, 1995). There have been situations where the interpreter refused to explain a terminal condition to a service user because of the strong community taboo and her own personal beliefs on this (Kaufert and Putsch, 1997).

In a study of migrant communities in an area of New South Wales, Australia, Norman (1996) found that the majority thought service users should not be directly informed of the seriousness of their illness because of the harm it could do. They believed the family should protect the service user from worry. However, when she asked if they themselves would wish to be told if they were terminally ill, the majority answered 'yes'. The reasons given were to get their affairs in order, to choose where to die, and to accept God's will. Hence a contradiction was revealed in her study.

The possibility of asking the service user whether he would want to have his medical situation explained to him directly or whether he would rather his family be informed of the situation, as a way of abiding by the duty to respect service user autonomy as well as acknowledging his cultural values, is not discussed. Medical interpreters who contravene cultural values in abiding by biomedical ethical practice can experience stressful situations.

Case example

A Bengali couple met with the paediatrician and interpreter. The doctor asked the interpreter to explain that the couple's baby daughter, who had suffered severe brain damage, was not responding to treatment and that the doctors wanted to raise with the parents the possibility of withdrawal of active treatment. The parents became extremely angry with the interpreter who had transgressed cultural beliefs in encouraging them to talk about the possibility they would agree to allow their child to die. The interpreter was able to explain that it was the doctor and not her saying these things and that it was the doctor's duty to discuss and involve them.

Failure to pursue embarrassing areas of questioning for fear of offence runs the risk of not offering the same quality of care to all service users. Failure to understand the service user does the same and is an issue of equal opportunity. Particular skills are therefore required.

The interpreter may be able to warn the health professional about areas that will cause offence so that some strategies for dealing with this can be discussed. This could include changing health professional or interpreter to one of the appropriate gender. The service user may feel offended by the interpreter who because they are of the same culture should know better than to ask such questions. They may get angry with the interpreter. One way to deal with this is to apologise that this may be a difficult area of enquiry and explain why the health professional thinks this information is important to obtain or relate.

Case example

A 20-year-old Turkish man is complaining of weight loss, flu-like symptoms, tiredness, and diarrhoea. The doctor wants to explore possible HIV infection.

DOCTOR: *Mustafa, have you ever had sex with another man?*
INTERPRETER: *Mustafa, have you ever had sex with another man?*
SERVICE USER: *What do you mean?*
INTERPRETER: *He says what do you mean?*
DOCTOR: *Have you ever slept with a man, have you ever had any form of sex with a man?*
INTERPRETER: *Have you ever slept with a man, have you ever had any form of sex with a man?*
SERVICE USER: *(hesitates) No.*
DOCTOR: *Do you know what I mean by safe sex?*
SERVICE USER: *(hesitates) Yes.*
INTERPRETER: *Well he says yes, but I think he is quite confused, could you perhaps explain why you are asking these questions?*

In this extract the interpreter is alerting the doctor to a problem. This may be due to genuine confusion, embarrassment or difficulty in talking about such matters. The interpreter may be suggesting a strategy that would help the service user to talk.

Open questions encourage a service user to talk and give them a lot of leeway e.g. 'Tell me about . . .?'. In situations where service users are uncomfortable to talk about a subject or do not readily have the language because it is not a subject that is voiced, selected closed questions to obtain key information may be appropriate. Enlist the help of the interpreter. Is there a way of approaching difficult conversations in this culture? Is it better to ask the questions in a straightforward manner or to comment on the difficulty, apologise, explain the importance and then ask the questions? Certain cultures may favour directness or indirectness in speech. The other side to this is the service users' fears of causing offence. These may override their ability to say no, disagree or indicate they don't understand. People may appear to agree when in fact they are displaying deference. It can be difficult to get accurate answers.

Leading questions and those which anticipate the answer 'yes' are particularly hazardous. Phrasing questions to expect the answer 'no' is one approach to increase accuracy. Checking with the interpreter if the response seems inaccurate and then modifying the approach can be helpful.

Working effectively with an interpreter

The key to working effectively is a trusting partnership, having confidence in the training, knowing the working methods, being clear about the code of conduct and understanding boundaries (Primary Care Support Force, 1996). A willingness to discuss improvements and raise any problems with the way of working together is important.

Interpreters in primary care may work with the same team of health professionals and are often able to establish a good working relationship as part of the team. Hospital settings may offer less consistency but any opportunity to meet before consultations and discuss afterwards how you worked together should promote collaboration.

Pre-consultation meeting between interpreter and health professional

Discuss your needs, hopes and any concerns about working with them which it would be useful to air. Invite their own views. It helps if the interpreter knows your objectives for the consultation and that you have checked her understanding of particular terms and concepts.

Discuss with the interpreter which style of interpretation to use. Should she translate every word or summarise your main points and is she free to ask the service user questions directly to clarify an issue? How will you know what she is doing?

It is better if the interpreter translates the service user's own words rather than paraphrasing or adjusting them into professional jargon. This gives a better sense of the service user's organisation of thought, level of understanding, concepts and emotional state, which is important information especially in the mental health interview. The interpreter should tell you whatever the service user says even if it sounds silly or embarrassing.

Encourage the interpreter to refrain from inserting her own interpretations or ideas or leaving out information that is thought irrelevant. Welcome her active involvement with you when she identifies problems. Encourage her to ask if she doesn't understand words you use, tell you if she needs to use explanations when there is no parallel expression for the one you use, let you know if what you are asking is culturally inappropriate, and tell you if she feels the service user is misunderstanding or giving an inaccurate reply.

Pre-consultation meeting between interpreter and service user

It is useful for the interpreter to meet the service user beforehand, however briefly, and begin to make a relationship, help put the service user at ease and find out something of the service user's educational level, attitudes towards health and health care. This can help the interpreter in gauging the depth and type of information and explanation that will be needed in a specific interview. It can also enhance the collaborative nature of interactions between interpreters, health workers and service users by establishing effective rapport (Hutton and Webb, 1993). The interpreter can explain her role and reassure the service user about confidentiality. She can indicate that anything the service user tells her will be conveyed to the health professional, so the service user can decide if there are things he does not want to say.

The bilingual consultation

Some guidelines for conducting the consultation are as follows;

- Preparation. Seating arrangements can be made before the service user and interpreter enter the room. Some recommend a triangle with the interpreter closer to the service user, others sit the interpreter to the side and slightly behind the service user to allow the health professional and service user closer contact. Ask the interpreter for the correct order and pronunciation of the service user's name.
- Welcome the service user by name, smile and shake hands if appropriate.
- Look at and speak to the service user not the interpreter. Speak as if you expect the service user to understand as he or

she may well be able to understand some of what you say. Don't speak pidgin English.

- Use a positive tone that conveys interest in the service user and take care not to raise your voice or use a tone which may feel patronising.
- Monitor the effect of your non-verbal behaviour such as eye contact and modify if necessary.
- Use direct speech if possible. Use active rather than passive form of verbs.
- Use clear statements planned in advance with language appropriate for the interpreter and expect to spend some time with the interpreter.
- Speak in short units of speech. Avoid long and complex explanations without a break. Indicate changes in direction.
- Allow the interpreter time to explain.
- Avoid technical or professional jargon and abbreviations.
- Avoid colloquialisms, slang, idiomatic expressions, similes, metaphors and indefinite phrases. Be careful with examples or analogy.
- Repeat information more than once. Always give the reason for treatment or prescription.
- Ask for feedback from the service user. This helps to check the service user's understanding and accuracy of translation. Ask the service user to repeat instructions or whatever has been communicated in his own words with translator facilitating.
- Ask for feedback on feelings, e.g. 'How do you feel about what I have told you?'
- Listen and watch the service user throughout to check for non-verbal communication of facial expressions, voice intonations, gestures and body movements. Although there may be cultural variations you may be able to check this asking e.g. 'Are you worried?' etc.
- Use empathy, acknowledgement and legitimation.
- Ask the interpreter to comment on non-verbal elements, the fullness of the service user's understanding and any culturally sensitive or culturally specific issues. This is likely to be particularly important in interpreting appropriate or inappropriate behaviour, and demeanour in the area of mental health. What would be the norm in one culture may seem inappropriate in another.

- Inevitably such an interview will take longer and patience is required. The interpreter may need to use longer explanatory phrases. Observing the service user and interpreter may however provide useful time to formulate ideas and further questions.

Meeting afterwards

After the consultation the interpreter can give her impressions of the service user and any cultural considerations. She may be able to add other information which she could not at the time. Discuss any difficulties about the process of interpretation and whether you were able to establish a relationship with the service user or whether you felt excluded. Ask the interpreter whether she had any problems with the interaction, with your own behaviour or with the service user. Identify together any ways it could be improved for the service user's sake and fulfilment of the functions in the consultation.

Concerns that health workers may have about working with interpreters

Doctors who work closely with interpreters report that this enables them to form a relationship with a service user which would not otherwise be the case and that they can get to know and understand their service users and the community (Primary Care Support Force, 1996). The working relationship that health professionals have with medical interpreters and the respect they have for them as fellow professionals would seem to be essential to discuss some of the concerns which sometimes arise.

- *Distortion*: Health workers may be concerned that interpreters are not translating but interpreting and putting in their own words or ideas. They may fail to understand a concept or term and use a word with other meaning. Interpreters could be leaving out something by accident or intention which changes the meaning. Long conversations with short translations make health professionals particularly nervous. Interpreters should be faithful to the speaker's intent whilst needing some flexibility about language, explanation and special needs.
- *Giving advice*: Inevitably interpreters will acquire knowledge of health services and medicine. The boundaries of what information they tell service users and what information should be

dealt with by the health professional may not always be clear and will depend very much on context. For example a trained medical interpreter working in an ante-natal clinic may do a screening interview and give health advice to a woman before she sees a doctor. Any uncertainty about giving advice needs to be discussed between the interpreter and health professional.

- *Whose agenda?*: At its extreme, the fear that interpreters may be working to an agenda and not translating accurately is a concern clinicians express. This can also be a source of tension for interpreters. If the interpreter is using an advocacy role in supporting the service user's autonomy and self determination then she may be raising matters of importance to the service user, which in the normal course of a consultation and because of the power imbalance may not ordinarily be voiced by a service user. This could either be welcomed by the health professional or be experienced as challenging or distorting. It would be important to discuss this with the interpreter who may be finding it difficult to raise the service user's concerns when the health professional seems not to want to hear them.

- *Tension between interpreter and service user*: The health worker may sense impatience or anger on the part of the interpreter. It may appear that the service user is being told off and that his words are not being translated. The interpreter may feel embarrassed or disapproving of the service user's behaviour, demands and coping methods. In instances where the interpreter speaks the same language but comes from a different social or cultural group from the service user there may be inherent tension between communities. Another possibility is that the prosodic features of tone of voice, stress, pauses or interruptions and pace of speech are suggesting conflict but are merely a difference in linguistic convention. Find out what the problem is, if the interpreter is angry, why and whether it is possible to resolve it.

What to do if you think there are problems with interpretation

Starting from the position of good intent these are all matters that should be discussed with the interpreter. It helps if there is already a relationship of respect, trust and collaboration.

UNIVERSITY COLLEGE LIBRARY CORK

It may be difficult to tell if things are going wrong and why but if you have concerns you may choose to stop the interview, ask the interpreter to explain to the service user that you need to discuss specific things with her and try to find out what the problem is. Alternatively have a discussion after the interview.

Training implications

Training with medical interpreters has revealed important role conflicts which they can sometimes experience in their work (Kaufert and Putsch, 1997). There would appear to be very little training of health professionals in how to work with interpreters but it is obvious that these are shared issues, which would benefit both sides to be able to explore and consider. This has the potential for not only improving consultations but also for recognising some of the conflicts that are not readily resolved through communication.

Discussion of how interpreters and health professionals work together with service users can help to promote good working practices and a collaborative approach to care. Training involving videotaping of consultations, with service users' consent, can be tremendously helpful in learning about the effect of different behaviours on achieving the goals of the consultation. Role-playing of consultations, if done in the spirit of constructive discovery together and watching how health professionals and interpreters work with service users can enhance working practices. The interpreter's role is considerably greater than one of language translation and if health professionals are able to work together utilising their skills and knowledge this will promote fulfilment of the goals in a consultation for both service users and providers.

References

Bird, J. and Cohen-Cole, S. A. (1990) 'The Three Function Model of the medical interview'. In M. S. Hale (ed.), *Advances in Psychosomatic Medicine*. Basel: Karger, vol. 20, pp. 65–88.

Blochliger, C., Tanner, M., Hatz, C. and Junghanss, T. (1997) 'Asylum seekers and refugees in ambulatory health care: communication between physician and service user (in German)'. *Schweiz Rundsch Med. Prax.*, 86 (19): 800–10.

Bochner, S. (1982) *Cultures in Contact: Studies in Cross-cultural Inter-action*. Oxford: Pergamon.

Boreham, P. and Gibson, D. (1978) 'The informative process in private medical consultations: a preliminary investigation'. *Social Science and Medicine*, 12: 409–416.

Brislin, R. and Yoshida, T. (1994) *Intercultural Communication Training: An Introduction*. London: Sage, pp. 85–87.

Carrese, J. A. and Rhodes, L. A. (1995) 'Western bioethics on the Navajo Reservation, benefit or harm'. *Journal of American Medical Association*, 274 (10): 826–9.

Chaturvedi, N., Rai, H. and Ben-Shlomo, Y. (1997) 'Lay diagnosis and health-care seeking behaviour for chest pain in south Asians and Europeans'. *Lancet*, 350 (9091): 1578–83.

Cunningham, C. and Davis, H. (1985) *Working with Service Users: Frameworks for Collaboration*. Milton Keynes: Open University Press.

Davis, H. and Fallowfield, L. (1990) *Counselling and Communication in Health Care*. Chichester: John Wiley and Sons, pp. 13–19.

Doyal, L. (1996) 'Consent for surgical treatment'. In R. M. Kirk, A. O. Mansfield and J. Cochrane (eds), *Clinical Surgery in General*. London: Churchill Livingstone, Chapter 11.

Engel, G. L. (1977) 'The need for a new medical model: a challenge for biomedicine'. *Science*, 196: 129–36.

Fuller, J. H. S. and Toon, P. D. (1988) *Medical Practice in a Multicultural Society*. Oxford: Butterworth-Heinemann, Chapter 2.

General Medical Council (1998) *Duties of a Doctor*. London: General Medical Council.

Gill, P., Scrivener, G., Lloyd, D. and Dowell, T. (1995) 'The effect of service user ethnicity on prescribing rates'. *Health Trends*, 27 (4): 111–113.

Hardt, E. J. (1995) 'The bilingual interview and medical interpretation'. In M. Lipkin Jr., S. M. Putnam and A. Lazare (eds), *The Medical Interview: Clinical Care, Education and Research*. London: Springer.

Hornberger, J. C., Gibson, C. D. Jr., Wood, W., Dequeldre, C., Corso, I., Palla, B. and Bloch, D. A. (1996) 'Eliminating language barriers for non-English-speaking service users'. *Med. Care*, 34 (8): 845–56.

Hornberger, J., Itakura, H. and Wilson, S. R. (1997) 'Bridging language and cultural barriers between physicians and service users'. *Public Health Rep.*, 112 (5): 410–7.

Hutton, D. C. and Webb, T. (1993) 'Information transmission in bilingual, bicultural contexts: a field study of community health nurses and interpreters'. *J. Community Health Nurs.*, 10 (3): 137–47.

Jackson, J. C., Rhodes, L. A., Inui, T. S. and Buchwald, D. (1997) 'Hepatitis B among Kmer. Issues of translation and concepts of illness'. *J. Gen. Intern. Med.*, 12 (5): 292–8.

Kaufert, J. M. and Koolage, W. W. (1984) 'Role conflict among "culture brokers": The experience of native Canadian medical interpreters', *Social Science and Medicine*, 18 (3): 283–6.

Kaufert, J. M. and Putsch, R. W. (1997) 'Communication through interpreters in healthcare: ethical dilemmas arising from differences in class, culture, language, and power'. *The Journal of Clinical Ethics*, 8 (1): 71–87.

Language Line Guide for Interpreters. Swallow House, 11–21 Northdown St, London, N1 9BN. E-mail: LanglineUK@aol.com.

Levinson, W., Roter, D.L., Mullooly, J.P., Dull, V.T. and Frankel, R.M. (1997) 'The relationship with malpractice claims among primary care physicians and surgeons'. *JAMA*, 277: 553–9.

Maguire, P. (1984) 'Communication skills and service user care'. In A. Steptoe and A. Matthews (eds), *Health Care and Human Behaviour*. London: Academic Press.

McWhinney, I. (1989) 'The need for a transformed clinical method'. In M. Stewart and D. Roter (eds), *Communicating with Medical Service Users*. Newbury Park, CA: Sage Publications, Chapter 1.

Marcos, L. R. (1979) 'Effects of interpreters on the evaluation of psycho-pathology in non-English speaking service users'. *Am. J. Psychiatry*, 136: 171–4.

Norman, C. (1996) 'Breaking bad news: consultations with ethnic communities'. *Australian Family Physician*, 25 (10): 1583–7.

Novack, D. H. (1995) 'Therapeutic aspects of the clinical encounter'. In M. Likpkin, S. M. Putnam and A. Lazare (eds), *The Medical Interview; Clinical Care, Education and Research*. New York: Springer, Chapter 3.

Primary Care Support Force (1996) 'More than Language'. A videotape of 'Working with Bi-Lingual advocates in Primary Care'. 40 Eastbourne Terrace, London, W2 3QR.

Quereshi, B. (1988) 'Ethnic gaps to bridge in the consultation'. *Geriatric Medicine*, August.

Randall-David, E. (1989) *Strategies for Working with Culturally Diverse Communities and Service users*. Washington, DC: The Association for the Care of Children's Health.

Roter, D. (1979) 'Altering service user behaviour in interaction with providers'. In D. Osborne, M. Gruneberg and J. Eiser (eds), *Research in Psychology and Medicine*. London: Academic Press, vol. 2.

Szasz, T. and Hollander, M. (1956) 'A contribution to the philosophy of medicine: the basic models of the doctor–service user relationship'. *Archives of Internal Medicine*, 97: 585–92.

Todd, A. D. and Fisher, S. (1993) *The Social Organisation of Doctor–Service User Communication*, 2nd edn. New Jersey: Ablex Publishing Corporation.

Tuckett, D., Boulton, M., Olsen, C. and Williams, A. (1985) *Meetings between Experts: An Approach to Sharing Ideas in the Consultation.* London: Tavistock.

Waitzkin, H. (1985) 'Information giving in medical care'. *J. Health Soc. Behav.*, 26: 81–101.

Chapter 3

Training issues for interpreters

Rachel Tribe with Marsha Sanders

Introduction

This chapter will discuss the importance of training for interpreters and those working alongside them. Training is vital if the service user is to receive an optimum service and clinicians are to make the best use of the opportunities afforded them by working with interpreters. Many clinicians feel very anxious about working with interpreters and this can easily affect the dynamics of the consultation and the service offered to the service user. An interpreter is frequently asked to undertake an extremely complex and sophisticated job, often interpreting words that may carry a lot of resonance and responsibility for the service user, but with little training on the complexities of the task. The interpreter's contribution to the team needs to be recognised. Without the interpreter, the service user may not be able to access treatment and most importantly the service user may feel very vulnerable and exposed having 'lost their own voice', and needing to rely on another person to relay all their health concerns. These anxieties can be exacerbated in a mental health context about which most societies have taboos or worries, and an individual may also have personal fears about the implications of how they or a family member is feeling or behaving. Training for clinicians and interpreters on working together in mental health can prove extremely helpful and improve the service offered to clients considerably. The department, agency and clinician may benefit also from obtaining access to another way of looking at mental health and any associated cultural or religious views, rather than simply assuming that the western way is the only way.

The chapter will consider what kind of training might be most useful for clinicians and interpreters. It will then review national training available for interpreters in Britain. Finally it will move on to make some suggestions about what kind of small scale training might benefit both interpreters and clinicians, and how agencies might consider setting this up. Finally the chapter incorporates some briefing guidelines for clinicians or agencies using interpreters. The author believes that training can be extremely beneficial for all concerned. It can help agencies consider issues of racism, stereotyping, and western health beliefs, as well as improving the agencies' clinical practice in the process.

Training and qualifications for interpreters

Interpreters work in a number of settings. These contexts can be divided loosely into commercial, for example in banking or international business, socio-legal and health or welfare. In the latter context, the interpreter might assist an individual or their family in access to health, legal and social welfare services. This chapter will concern itself more specifically with training for interpreting in mental health contexts. Countries in parts of Scandinavia and the Antipodes have run interpretation courses for many years, however training and qualifications for interpreters have not yet become established within the mainstream in Britain. This lack of regulated training courses and qualifications has had an adverse effect on the status and professional identity and role of interpreters, with employing organisations being unable to verify the level of expertise and training which an interpreter holds. It has meant there are no national or NHS guidelines or qualification points for interpreters who would like to enhance their skills and training. The author believes that if the role and contribution of interpreters is to be optimised, a national framework of qualifications needs to be established although work on this is starting, as described later in the chapter. This may also encourage employing organisations to further recognise the contribution of interpreters.

Two organisations have started to accredit training courses. The best known is probably the Institute of Linguists, which follows the linguistic model of interpreting and where many of the students are working in the commercial sector. They accredit a range of qualifications including Diploma in Public Service Interpreting (DPSI), within the areas of health, law and public services or local government. The final examination is said to be on a par with an undergraduate degree. It is available in some adult and continuing education institutions throughout Britain, or as a distance learning option nation-wide. A range of courses are also run by individual colleges and universities. Unfortunately some organisations' emphasis on academic qualifications at the point of entry appears to restrict access to many interpreters who may be bilingual and steeped in two cultures, but who do not possess formal British educational qualifications.

The Open College Federation has a somewhat different perspective; their courses are more orientated towards a client-centred community advocacy approach and operate nationally. The London Open College Network (LOCN) in collaboration with a consortium of community interpreter trainers has established a course for interpreters. This consists of an introductory course comprising compulsory core and optional units that can be assessed at three different levels. In addition to the core units of community interpreting skills, there is a unit on developing research skills and compiling a bilingual glossary. Other units may be made available to provide a more specialised course. A variety of assessment methods are used, including self and peer evaluation, evaluation by external language assessors and written assignments. As these courses are oriented towards interpreters working for their communities within health and welfare, they also touch upon social and community work, the importance of understanding cultural, religious and racial variables, racism, discrimination and issues of power and empowerment.

It is difficult for agencies and clinicians to determine who is a highly qualified or experienced interpreter and who is a beginner, as well as meaning that interpreters have no established career path. In addition this may convey a message that anyone who is bilingual can act as an interpreter. This can be a dangerous assumption particularly in a mental health context. Apart from linguistic skills, interpreters may also act as cultural brokers, link-workers or cultural consultants for service users and clinicians (these are all explained earlier, see Chapter 1, pp. 17 and 18). This is important if the contribution of different explanatory beliefs about health is to be integrated into an understanding of the service user's presentation and possibly their subsequent treatment. Recent developments in this field have lead to the possibility of developing a national qualification which fits within the National Vocational Qualifications (NVQ) framework. This is being discussed by the Institute of Linguists, the Register of Public Service Interpreters and the Languages National Training Organisation (LNTO). The latter agency represents the Government's national strategy for language. At the current time this qualification is only available at the highest NVQ level which is level 5. This equates with a postgraduate or professional qualification. It is hoped that, in time, NVQs will be available at the other four (1–4) levels. This should go a long way to recognising the important work of interpreters by ensuring there is a clear raft of qualifications which fits into a national qualifications framework.

Interpreters and clinicians require training related to working together if the service user is to obtain a good service. The author can remember fighting a very difficult battle to get the role and contribution of interpreters recognised in an agency working exclusively with refugees, where many of the service users required interpreters. Some of the clinicians (paid) felt that it should remain a 'Cinderella' service, with the interpreters undertaking their work on a voluntary basis or being paid a minimum amount. The reasons given were that they were not professionals and had no recognised training. The cycle therefore became recursive and increasingly difficult to break. After a long struggle this agency finally changed its position and now views interpreters and bicultural workers as having a central role to play in its clinical work. It is important to realise that there may be a perceived power imbalance between the participants in the clinical interview, issues of ascribed power and racist or dominant beliefs, which may need consideration and attention. In addition two of the three members of the triad may feel excluded from the consultation. Issues of transference may also be present.

Apart from training at the national level as already described, it can also be done at the agency or health authority level. For this to happen first a generic training course on the roles, responsibilities and skills required of interpreters would need to be undertaken. A module on mental health could be included in this or a further course specifically on mental health could be run. Either way, it would need to start with definitions of mental health, well-being and illness, and the importance of context and meaning; the differences between learning difficulties and mental health being clearly identified. Participants' contributions should form a large part of the course otherwise, if this were not the case, the inequalities of racism and western health beliefs might be replicated. It is also important to place the course at the appropriate level, which will vary depending on the objectives of the course. The aim should be to ensure that interpreters have enough information to be able to do as good a job as possible. The aim is not to try and train pseudo-clinicians; interpreters have their own profession.

Different agencies will have different requirements. Some may find they require interpreters infrequently, while others that they need to have a regular team. Some agencies will wish interpreters to have a good understanding of different therapeutic approaches, while others will feel a briefing and de-briefing at the beginning and end of the session is sufficient. One agency may believe it is important for interpreters to understand about traumatic reactions and basic diagnostic categories, another that this is irrelevant and should remain within the remit of the clinician only. Whatever the arrangements, interpreters are often privy to extremely sensitive information and they will need training and support to help them hold this information.

Your agency may wish to include some or all of the following modules in a training course for interpreters working within mental health:

- A general introduction to mental health provision within the health trust, and the particular agency in which the interpreter is likely to be based.
- A brief explanation of what the different mental health professionals do, for example what are the major differences between a psychiatrist, psychologist, psychiatric nurse, psychotherapist, and psychiatric social worker.
- An explanation of concepts such as working as part of a multi-disciplinary team.
- An overview of how working therapeutically may differ from undertaking an assessment.
- Discussions around what mental well-being/health and mental illness may mean, including issues of causation incorporating different cultural and theoretical views about this.
- A very brief overview of the Mental Health Act and other relevant legislation. The exact content is likely to vary depending upon the agency and the interpreter's requirements.
- An overview of the most common presenting problems that an interpreter is likely to come across. For example, if the interpreter is likely to be working mostly with asylum-seekers, this might include depression and traumatic and somatic reactions.

- A session based on dealing with difficult interpreting situations in mental health. For example when the service user tells the interpreter something and then asks the interpreter not to tell the clinician, or when a service user is psychotic. A mixture of discussion and role-plays around these issues may be most helpful.

- Issues relating to boundaries should also be covered. Interpreters are often put under considerable pressure by clients and clinicians to take on tasks that go beyond their remit. A service user who is unable to access services because they are unfamiliar with the English language would be more likely to try and make the most of having access to someone who not only speaks both languages fluently, but is familiar with how the different systems work and may be of invaluable help to them. Exactly where the boundaries are to be established needs careful consideration. For example, some clinicians view interpreters as an asset to the therapeutic session and may negotiate with the interpreter for them to play an active role in the consultation and to share knowledge and understanding. On other occasions, it may be appropriate for the interpreter merely to interpret the clinician's words in the session and not be available to the service user or clinician outside this session. How the role is to be negotiated and managed needs to be discussed by the clinician and interpreter before a session begins and before the service user enters the room. Any training course needs to consider the possible roles and how these might be negotiated.

The author has found that the use of role-plays can bring some of these issues alive and make what might be a rather dry subject, relevant and alive. In addition the agency should have written guidelines and perhaps a contract that the interpreters may be asked to adhere to or to sign.

- Ethical considerations for interpreters and familiarity with any ethical codes established by the relevant employing agency.

Confidentiality is another area of vital importance particularly within the mental health arena. Mental health professionals have usually undergone a rigorous training that has incorporated the importance of confidentiality within the mental health team. However, interpreters may believe that talking to others may help them obtain information that might be useful to the service user.

The importance of total confidentiality needs discussing on any training course within this area. Linked to this is the need for proper support and supervision for interpreters, as for any staff working within mental health (as described in Tribe, 1999). Given that interpreters frequently come from the linguistic community they are representing, they may come under enormous pressure to share information with other members of the community. In addition they may also know the client or their family before the session. If this is the case the clinician and interpreter needs to decide whether this is appropriate, or if they will seek another interpreter.

- Lines of accountability: different agencies may have different policies on this, it may be to the head of the interpreting team or it may be the clinician the interpreter is working with. This will require clarification.

If there is more than one interpreter of a language they may find it useful to discuss how they are translating particular words, especially those which do not translate directly or which have a somewhat ambivalent meaning in either language. After running a support and supervision group for interpreters at one agency, it was decided that it would be useful to have a medical or psychology dictionary in each consulting room for interpreters to consult. Unless someone has worked within mental health in the two countries or has had a lot of dealings with mental health agencies, there are likely to be specialist professional languages with which they have never come into contact. Establishing an organisational culture where this is recognised, rather than a culture where an interpreter is made to feel an unwelcome addition or incompetent if they are not familiar with specialist language will improve the service to the service user considerably. If an interpreter does not feel comfortable asking for clarification or being able to acknowledge being unfamiliar with the exact meaning of specialist language, the service user may receive a second-rate service. It is important to include interpreters in any regular induction courses that your agency runs. As well as having an integrating function, this would provide the interpreter with useful information about the organisational culture, the ethos of the organisation, what it is trying to achieve, and what exactly its mission is and the parameters thereof. Interpreters may hold a number of different roles, as described by Raval (Chapter 1) and Baylav (Chapter 4). These have been described elsewhere in the book, they will not be re-iterated again. Suffice to say that any training course should cover all of these and detailed discussions about their advantages and disadvantages. As professional interpreters they also have the right to turn down work or assignments that they feel are not compatible with their training and expertise. Agencies may wish to consider issuing best practice guidelines to interpreters and mental health practitioners, to ensure that the issues previously discussed in this chapter are clearly expressed and reflect an organisational culture where these issues have been considered and their importance noted.

Conclusion

In summary, the author believes that nationally recognised qualifications need to be established if the work of interpreters is to receive the recognition it deserves. This does not mean that individual agencies cannot do a lot to ensure that their interpreters are trained and recognised as important members of the clinical team. Any training will ideally involve clinicians and interpreters receiving training together as part of the organisation's regular training and professional development opportunities. This is likely to enhance the service offered to service users requiring interpreters, as well as ensuring that different views about mental health and culture are adequately integrated and respected within clinical practice. Guidelines on working with interpreters and best practice need to be developed by each agency in conjunction with their interpreters, to ensure that service users receive the best service possible and that their inability to communicate in English does not preclude them accessing appropriate mental health services. One set of possible guidelines is given below; these are likely to require fine-tuning and amending to ensure they fit the agencies' requirements.

BRIEF GUIDELINES ON WORKING WITH INTERPRETERS

Introduction

Communicating through a third person is a challenging task; the recognition of this simple fact can go a long way towards planning for a first meeting using an interpreter.

This can be assisted by:

- The provision of trained and experienced interpreters with on-going support from either an organisation or individual.
- The provision of effective guidelines and appropriate training for health professionals who use interpreters.

The following information should help each clinician to develop his or her own effective way of working with professional interpreters.

Booking an interpreter

This may be done through an interpreting agency such as Essential Interpreters and Translators International (EITI) or through your agencies' own panel of interpreters. Sometimes service users are reluctant to admit their need for an interpreter. It is the clinician's responsibility to discuss with the service user or relevant others if an interpreter would assist the consultation.

Before making a booking

Find out what is the service user's first language and if he or she speaks any other languages fluently

Many people from ethnic groups speak two or more languages and the more languages they speak fluently, the more choice and flexibility there is to organise an appropriate interpreter. It is always preferable to use an interpreter who is proficient in the service user's first choice of language, particularly within mental health where the service user's exact meaning and intent may be extremely important.

Identify the dialect spoken

Most languages have several dialects. Do not assume that someone who speaks a language can speak it in all the dialects.

Suggest a time and place for the consultation, as well as several alternatives, in case the requested interpreter is not available on the original date

Agree the broad subject matter of the consultation

This is helpful in selecting an interpreter who is familiar with and has some training in mental health. It will also preclude an interpreter who may feel uncomfortable or anxious about working within mental health. As important, it helps to exclude interpreters who may have a special sensitivity to the subject matter. For instance, it might be inappropriate to expect someone believing that their family has been devastated by a family member who has been labelled as schizophrenic, to interpret for a service user with this diagnosis, or for a victim of organised violence or torture, who has themselves been tortured, to interpret for a service user seeking help for this atrocity.

Provide the interpreter with as much notice as possible

Other information to take into account

The nationality of the service user

Sharing a common language is often not sufficient for two people to communicate. Other factors such as culture and even political affiliations play a major role in influencing communication. It is often best to request an interpreter of the same nationality.

Gender and age

It may be helpful to match the gender and age of the interpreter to that of the service user.

Religion

As far as possible it is advisable to arrange an interpreter who, if not from the same religion as the service user, has a good understanding of his or her religion.

Time allowed for the interview

Since all conversation needs to be translated, give yourself at least double the time for a normal interview.

Double bookings

If other colleagues work with a particular service user make sure that the interpreter has not been booked by another clinician in the organisation for a consultation.

Future meetings

If you wish to use the same interpreter for a series of consultations make sure that you emphasise this at the time of the initial booking and provide a list of dates.

Points to consider

- The interpreter has to gain your service user's trust as well as your own. The most effective interpreter is one who behaves, acts and appears neutral. Do not expect a professional interpreter to take sides for any reason. Partiality, even if it has a positive effect in the short term, is unhelpful in the long run and may reduce or even destroy the service user's trust of both interpreter and health professional.
- Try not to leave the interpreter alone with the service user. Interpreters may be put under a great deal of pressure in these circumstances.
- Do not expect all meanings and thoughts to be conveyed perfectly. Language is not a set of formulas and words with accurate associated meanings, but rather a whole way of life and conceptualisation. Words do not necessarily have precise equivalents in other languages. It may be that a sentence with 4 English words takes 20 words to interpret. Therefore do not become impatient if the interpreter takes longer to translate than you expect.
- You may need to slow down your pace; remember the interpreter has to remember what you have said, translate it and then convey it to the service user. If you speak for too long, the interpreter may be hard pressed to remember the first part of what you said. Conversely, if you speak in too short bursts, you may find that your speech becomes fragmented and you lose the thread of what you are saying. You will find, that with open communication and trust, a natural rhythm becomes established, which everyone feels comfortable with.

- Try to spend some time considering all the implications of working with a third party, the interpreter. You may find it helpful to discuss this with an interpreter and with colleagues who have experience of working with interpreters.

Before the consultation

Additional preparation is required before a meeting where an interpreter is to be used takes place. Remember that having an interpreter as a mediator makes you dependent on another person and this will alter the dynamics of all the interactions during the interview. Therefore you need to be extremely clear about what the objectives of the meeting are, and what strategy you will need to use in order to control the meeting.

It is of vital importance to arrange a pre-meeting session with the interpreter, preferably immediately before the actual interview. Spending 10 minutes in this way beforehand may save you hours in the long run. This is especially crucial if any of the participants in the consultation have not met before.

Use this time to:

- Familiarise the interpreter with yourself, your agency and its goals.
- Clarify the objectives of the meeting.
- Consider how you will manage a three-way consultation. You may wish to move the furniture around before the service user arrives; there are several schools of thought on this. Some people believe a triangular-shaped arrangement works best, where everyone can see everyone else. Others, particularly in Australia, believe that the interpreter should sit behind the service user and act merely as the service user's voice, with all speech being delivered in the first person singular.

Ask the interpreter to update you on cultural matters relevant to the service user. The more you know about someone's culture, the better you can communicate with him or her and the more you can prevent disappointing results. Your awareness of cultural, religious and behavioural aspects of the service user plays a positive and influential role in your approach and decision-making. The interpreter is not only a linguist, but also a source of cultural information, and using him or her for this purpose also gives him or her more confidence and a sense of usefulness. In addition this will help the interpreter to relax in his or her role and help to create a comfortable atmosphere for the interview. You may also gain valuable knowledge to inform you better about the forthcoming meeting. Review some of the key words relating to the case with the interpreter and make sure he or she understands them and associates with them the same meaning as you do. For example the word trauma or counselling may not exist in another language, or they may carry a very different valence to that which the clinician intended. Time spent reviewing this will be a useful investment in the longer term.

Depending on the nature of the interview and its objectives, you may choose a method of interpreting that best suits the occasion. This needs to be discussed with the interpreter in advance. For instance, you may only want to be told the gist of issues discussed, as opposed to every detail, thus giving some liberty to the interpreter to summarise the translations. Alternatively, you may need the entire discussion to be translated word-for-word. In any event do not expect the interpreter to do your job. In order to establish some facts you may find it necessary to ask the service user a series of questions. The structure and order of these questions should be constructed by yourself and not by the interpreter, unless you agree to work in a different manner at the beginning.

When an interpreter is new to a case, always provide him or her with a brief case history relevant to the consultation. This information will help the interpreter to translate more accurately because he or she will be more aware of the overall picture of the service user's life. This additional awareness also allows the interpreter to know what to expect from the interview.

During the consultation

Allow some time for the interpreter and the service user to introduce themselves.

In spite of all preparations you often find that the service user is initially uneasy with the presence of an interpreter. This could be caused by cultural pressures leading to over-defensiveness, anger or even a sense of shame and embarrassment.

You may find it useful in these circumstances to reintroduce the interpreter in your own words with the help of the interpreter. Confirm that the interpreter is a professional doing his or her job.

Stress that the interpreter is independent and is present to facilitate communication between you and the service user. Clarify that he or she is not there to make any evaluations, and has no decision-making powers and is bound by the agency's confidentiality policy.

Try to avoid using specialist terminology unless it is essential. We often get too familiar with our organisation's and profession's specialist language and take it for granted that everyone else will understand it. This is difficult enough when dealing with people who understand English perfectly, but when communicating through an interpreter the problem multiplies. By using straight-forward language, you can reduce the possibility of misunder-standings and misinterpretations. For example, if you refer to OCD or PTSD this may have no meaning to a service user, who may feel unable to ask for clarification.

Avoid using proverbs and sayings. Many proverbs do not translate into other languages and any attempts to translate them results in misunderstandings. A good rule to follow is that what-ever does not make literal sense will not translate well into another language.

Provide sufficient breaks during the interview. Even a few occa-sional seconds of silence is extremely helpful. Interpreting is exhausting. Both you and the service user have the opportunity to rest your minds for a few moments while the interpreter is trans-lating into the other language. The interpreter, however, is con-stantly either listening or interpreting.

While in the presence of the service user, avoid discussing issues with the interpreter that do not require interpretation. This usually leads to tension between the interpreter and the service user. Keep these matters for after the meeting. If it is absolutely necessary to deviate from this rule make sure you explain this before the inter-view begins.

After the consultation

Spending a few minutes with the interpreter after each meeting can prove to be very fruitful. Make the interpreter comfortable enough to give his or her impression of the meeting. You will often find that interpreters, relieved from the pressure of the interview, can provide useful observations and information. You can also use the time to ask the interpreter to clarify cultural issues and seek meaning for points that were not clear during the meeting. Welcome criticism of yourself, even if you do not agree with the interpreter. This may help you to understand how people from the particular culture of your service user perceive you and the way you approach your work. Avoid over-generalisation.

Discuss your own observations of the interpreter's performance. If you have serious doubts about the interpreter's conduct, make sure you provide this feedback to his or her organisation after having discussed it with the interpreter. This is crucial in the development and improvement of the quality of the service provided by your organisation.

Acknowledgement

The author would like to acknowledge the contribution of Essential Interpreters and Translators International (EITI) in compiling these guidelines.

References and possible useful resources

Hoffman, L. (1989) *Lost in Translation*. London: William Heineman.

Raval, H. (1996) 'A systemic perspective on working with interpreters'. *Clinical Child Psychology and Psychiatry*, 1(1): 29–43.

Shackman, J. (1985) *The right to be understood. A handbook on working with interpreters*. London: The National Extension College.

Tribe, R. (1999) 'Bridging the gap or damming the flow? Using interpreters/bicultural workers when working with refugee clients, many of whom have been tortured'. *British Journal of Medical Psychology*, 72: 567–576.

Chapter 4

Issues of language provision in health care services

Akgul Baylav

Introduction

Effective communication is necessary for the provision of good quality health care as it enables a helpful process in being able to meet the service user's needs. However, due to language and cultural differences many service users do not receive health services on a par with their English-speaking compatriots. Language differences can be excluding in terms of service users not being able to access relevant information about services, not being able to communicate needs, not being understood, and not being able to feel empowered in determining the types of services that are provided. For example, there still remain discrepancies across health services with regards to the quality and availability of basic service information that is translated into different languages. Potential service users need to know about services that exist locally, what is involved in being able to access these, have their health needs identified and met, and be able to have an equal say in negotiating their health needs with service providers. Whilst many health care services are addressing issues of inequality and access for ethnic minority service users, there is a need for a continuous process change if all communities are going to benefit from the health care provision that is available.

The need for interpreters

Experienced and qualified interpreters facilitate a process of communication that is mutually beneficial to the service user and the service provider. Each person is likely to experience a sense of having been understood when the process of interpreting has taken place in a constructive manner. Though consultations with an interpreter take longer they are still likely to be more cost-effective in the long run, as they will enable more accurate diagnoses to be made, and therefore more effective treatment to be planned and implemented.

In the NHS, health care services are provided across different service provision contexts in primary, secondary, and tertiary settings. Health care provision is aimed at both prevention and treatment. Interpreters play an important role in helping service users become aware of the health provision that is available, and thereby increasing the levels of access for members of the community who may not typically seek out health care. It is important that interpreters take on numerous roles such as bilingual worker, advocate, health advisor, and link-worker in order to meet the needs of the ethnic minority service users in a more comprehensive manner.

The types of roles that are taken on by interpreters

In this chapter the general term 'language support' will be used to refer to the work of community interpreters, bilingual link-workers/advocates, and translators working in health care settings. The main roles that interpreters usually take on are described below:

Advocate: Challenges discrimination, negotiates, gives advice and information to enable choice and informed decisions, supports and empowers the service user.

Link-worker: Offers befriending and information to service user, and provides cultural information to service providers.

Interpreter: Facilitates communication for service user (who may be in unfamiliar surroundings, speak little or no English, and feel vulnerable and powerless). Interpreters, community interpreters, link-workers and advocates help to bridge the gap of equality and power between service users and service providers.

Let us imagine a situation where a service user is unwell and goes to see a doctor. The service user is ill, feels fragile and vulnerable. He or she is not familiar with the system and surroundings, speaks little or no English and needs treatment. The doctor, from whichever ethnic background, is in his or her own surroundings and is knowledgeable and powerful. With no language support these two parties cannot speak to each other. They may attempt to communicate with gestures and signs, but this, even with the best of intentions, is prone to misunderstandings and frustrations.

Bring into this situation an interpreter. The two parties can at least talk to each other. But this does not necessarily mean that they can understand each other. If the service user knows what he or she needs, and is articulate and confident enough to express those needs, then a good interpreter may be sufficient to ensure access to the services. Access is also improved if the doctor or health care provider is aware of the service user's possible needs and can explore and deal with them through the use of sensitive and appropriate questions. However, this is a rare situation and often the communication gap remains.

A bilingual link-worker introduced into this situation will interpret for the service user, his or her carer/s, and for the health care providers involved. She (as link-workers are usually women) will also help shed some light on cultural issues for each service user. This will work in a situation without prejudice and discrimination. But usually interpreters and link-workers have a very limited brief and cannot go beyond it, especially when they experience or observe discrimination towards service users or communities.

In this case bilingual advocates are best placed to negotiate, not only on behalf of but also in partnership with the service users, and to challenge discrimination if and when necessary. Advocates can act independently of the health service providers and are accountable primarily to the service users and communities.

The alternative

In the absence of language support a number of possible outcomes are possible. These include:

1. The service user may be reluctant to use a service and not actually get to the service that he or she may need.
2. Service users may find themselves struggling to communicate their needs, as the service provider has not provided an interpreter. The chances of poor communication and misinformation will be higher, and the service user is likely to get a second rate service.

3. A service user may choose to take a relative or friend. This will bring with it issues of confidentiality, power imbalances, and the appropriateness of a relative being present during a medical or therapeutic consultation, and it will affect the extent to which a service user will feel able to discuss personal information with the clinician. It may set up unhelpful dynamics between a service user and their friend or relative. Children are often put into the position of having to interpret for their parents, and in most instances this places them in an inappropriate relationship with their parents.

4. Unofficial community interpreters may again make it difficult for service users (under certain circumstances) to feel able to discuss all their health or mental health needs in front of a member of their local community. Confidentiality issues need consideration. The community helper may not have the requisite skills or experience to interpret in specialised settings such as mental health.

For example, in hospitals, interpreters generally work in specialist services such as maternity or mental health, and their job finishes at the end of the consultation. They receive specialist training in the procedures and terminology of the service they are based in and feel confident in dealing with both the service users and service providers within it. In primary care however, interpreters have to deal with the service users as they come through the door. Each comes with a different issue, manifested in a variety of ways ranging from simple physical complaints to complex mental health problems. It would not be an exaggeration to say that a primary care interpreter's caseload is as varied as that of a GP. Furthermore, interpreters often get involved in the follow-up work because service users visit their family doctor or dentist throughout their lives.

Service users need information about the types of services that are available. They also need to be told about their rights and entitlements, given the necessary explanations in a sensitive manner to alleviate the anxiety and stress associated with their condition, and enabled to make informed choices in relation to the treatment and care they receive. Service users need to be reassured that they are being listened to and that the service provider will address their concerns properly.

Health care service providers also need information about the communities they serve. They need to know about the cultural background and the present lifestyles affecting the health and health care of their service users. They need to be reassured that the medical advice and information they offer is being accurately transmitted without being compromised. And just like some of their service users, they themselves need language support because they cannot communicate in their service users' language.

Service specifications

Service specifications are often referred to as purchasing tools. This is so because purchasers and commissioners of health services, having established and agreed their policy for language services and conducted the relevant needs' assessment research, are in a position to specify what kind of language support service would be appropriate to have in place within specific settings. Once established, the specifications can be amended through ongoing review and evaluation to allow for developing the services or changing the focus. Most health authorities now include elements of specifying language support services within their general quality specification. For example, this has included:

1. Identifying local community language needs.
2. Health authorities developing translation and information policies for ensuring the provision of comprehensive language support services.
3. Locality-based services: personal, face-to-face language support services, i.e. interpreting and bilingual advocacy are best provided from a local site, whether in the hospital, health centre or local office base. The advantages are familiarity with the service and service providers, as well as with the local communities and agencies, good facilities for referral to local networks or agencies for additional support, services being easily accessible and readily available (particularly in emergencies), and the provision of on-call support during office hours, outreach support at home when needed.
4. Dedicated sessions: these are sessions where language support is provided regularly for a specific group of service users. They are pre-arranged, preferably in consultation with the group they are aimed at, and are available to all who need language support in contact with that specific service, e.g. maternity, GP or dental services. This helps the service provider to concen-

trate on the needs of one specific group and arrange other language-based help as necessary (e.g. bilingual receptionists or setting up video showings in the waiting area). Consistency and predictability of support, i.e. knowing that an interpreter or bilingual advocate will be there at the session, will increase the uptake of the services and improve access for that specific service user group. It will also give the interpreters the chance to familiarise themselves with the specific terminology required within a particular setting. New opportunities will open up for preventative work too. Health promotion sessions for groups from the same community with similar ideas, lifestyles and concerns will not only furnish them with much needed information, but also with the opportunity to provide mutual support in the community long after the session is over. The waiting room area can be used to show videos and display health promotion/services information leaflets as appropriate.

5. Specialist services: these are sessions where language support is provided regularly within a specific service. The interpreters/ bilingual link-workers or advocates are based within the service (e.g. maternity, cardiovascular disease or diabetes), and work only with the users and providers of that service. This gives them a good working knowledge of specialist terminology and familiarity with the service, which helps to establish trust between themselves and users (both community members and providers of health services), and also establishes a continuity of service for them. In different specialist set-ups, the role of the language support provider may change focus to have:

- A health management function (e.g. maternity, cardio-vascular disease, diabetes)
- A counselling function (e.g. HIV/AIDS, haemoglobino-paties)
- A specialist function as in mental health settings.

6. Recruitment/retention/career development: different roles as described above, performed in different settings within health care services, make it imperative to clarify the role of the language support worker needed as this will affect the job description and person specification of the worker, as well as the staffing levels, and structure and management of the

services. These considerations highlight the need to hold training seminars devoted specifically to the issue of language-based services within health care settings with the aim of:

- Discussing and agreeing definitions of these services (interpreting/community interpreting/translating/link-working/bilingual advocacy/bilingual clinical service providers)
- Establishing quality standards for such services
- Developing informed and evidence-based clinical approaches
- Looking at organisational structures and management of such services
- Looking at training models for bilingual workers and other service providers working with them
- Identifying sources of funding
- Looking at the future of language support with health services

Models of interpreting

Different models of interpreting have been suggested as follows:

1. The linguistic model, including telephone interpreting: a free-lance interpreter is called in to enable communication between the service user and service provider without any direct input into the outcome of the consultation other than competent and accurate interpretation of the conversations. This model works well when service users know what they want, are articulate enough to express it and assertive enough to demand it.
2. The service provider team model: the interpreter or the bilingual link-worker is part of a service provider (often clinical) team and helps to improve the service uptake by members of ethnic minority communities.
3. The service user centred model: the interpreter acts as a bilingual advocate taking on the functions of support, providing information, challenging and negotiating on behalf of the service users. The service user determines the extent and direction of this support.

All of these models have advantages and disadvantages. Recent experience has shown that no one model can be employed to adequately address all the communication needs of service users and providers of health services. Provision should be made, as far as practically possible, for different models to coexist within each service in order to give service users a choice. In addition, the bilingual workers themselves should be trained in such a way that they can employ clinical models flexibly, be able to adopt different roles with confidence, and be able to work in a competent manner across different service settings and different service user circumstances.

Conclusion

There still remains a need for developing and implementing quality standards for the work of practitioners and interpreters working in the health service. To some extent these need to evolve out of joint training and working for interpreters and clinicians. Whilst good progress has been made in this area of work, there is still a long way to go in being able to provide equitable and good quality service provision for many service users who need the help of an interpreter to fully access health care provision.

Chapter 5

A day in the life of an interpreting service[1]

Fardis Nijad

Introduction

For most of us the gift of speech is so much a part of our daily lives that we take it completely for granted. We only become aware of it when something goes wrong. There is therefore a danger that we can undervalue this highly complex facility of the human brain. The creative tool of language allows us, if we pause to consider it, to communicate myriad ideas using finite grammar and vocabulary.

Sometimes communication may suffer an apparently minor breakdown because of an unknown word. We may, for example, come across an unfamiliar word but the solution is at hand. We have only to reach for the dictionary to find the definition and so bridge the gap in communication.

But can the dictionary always bridge that gap completely? No lexicographer, however learned or experienced, can build into his definition of a word, the wealth of individual connotations and experiences that it represents for the user. It is in the *use* that language comes alive, and that life is generated not only by the linguistic context, but by a range of other factors too.

A knife is not just a knife. To each of us, depending on our preconceptions and experiences, a knife can have different connotations. If you have recently accidentally cut your finger on a kitchen knife, the word 'knife' can immediately take your thoughts back to your painful experience. Even if two people have

---

[1] Please note that this chapter was written before the Balkan conflict and some of the terminology is now different.

had the same experience their reactions may vary depending on their past experiences and individual characteristics. One person may think of the incident and feel vulnerable, another may even re-experience the pain in the finger, whilst yet another may laugh off the incident. The interesting thing is that in conversation the speaker often does not know about the past experiences or personality of the listener. He or she uses a word in the context of his or her own experiences in relation to the referent.

Thus, whilst in the dictionary a word may have a precise definition, in everyday use it rarely represents an identical concept in the minds of all speakers. Rather it comes with attendant baggage of ideas associated with the user's past experiences. Just as a picnic basket usually contains food and drink and a variety of utensils, so we can assume that others enjoying the pleasures of dining alfresco will have sandwiches, fizzy drinks and a sharp knife in their basket. But whilst in one hamper the sandwiches may be made with a sliced white loaf, others may prefer wholemeal rolls, and in France there will surely be baguettes. This is before we even start to consider the fillings or the vintage of the champagne!

When we communicate verbally we do so effectively only to the extent that the contents of our 'picnic baskets' overlap, or when we remember that even the same items can take different forms.

Nevertheless most of us do manage to understand each other well in the majority of our everyday conversations. Difficulties arise more frequently when we talk about concepts. When we discuss thoughts or emotions we can often seem to be speaking the same language whilst in reality giving the same words different meanings. It is therefore no wonder that although we are frequently successful in effective communication with close friends, the more distant a person is from us the more difficulty we have. In fact the problem is aggravated if the other party is of a different gender, age, social class or religion, and especially if the person is from another culture altogether. And that is when the parties share the same first language.

If the first language of the person with whom we wish to communicate is different, we often call on the services of an interpreter. We usually assume (wrongly) that since the interpreter speaks both languages we can expect communication to go smoothly. We mistakenly expect the interpreter to overcome all of the above problems in addition to translating the actual words. In fact what may happen is that by using a third person we open up new possibilities for misunderstanding. The right interpreter on the other hand can facilitate communication, point out cultural factors, clarify important and ambiguous points, and overall make it possible for two people from different worlds to communicate the true meaning of their words. This requires not only linguistic and cultural knowledge, but as the above implies, an array of other skills.

An effective interpreter is one who is not only able to translate words, but who is also familiar with the likely contents of the 'picnic baskets' that the speaker and listener are carrying with them. The interpreter therefore needs a very good understanding of the speaker's circumstances, lifestyle and past experiences, and of the influence of factors such as gender and religious belief.

This may all sound like overkill. However, the more intensely ambiguous the subject matter is, the greater the need for that perfect interpreter. That is why it may be easy to find an interpreter who can translate a mathematical formula because maths does not contain feelings. Legal matters, by their nature, contain less ambiguity. A legal interpreter does of course require knowledge of legal jargon and access to specialist glossaries, but he or she would have a more sensitive task interpreting on a more intimate or psychologically-charged matter. And it becomes more complicated the further away we get from straightforward formulae. The number 'one' means the same thing in most languages. 'One plus one' likewise. But the word 'pain' has hundreds of meanings. 'Missing', 'hate', 'love', 'confused', 'relax', all these words are an open invitation to explore concepts and feelings. If interpreting for an accountant is the least ambiguous, interpreting for a mental health service user is at the opposite end of the spectrum.

In such a case, the therapist's first job is to assess the service user. Through training and experience the therapist can identify patterns of thought by listening to him or her. The complex aspects of communication involving culture, symbolic gestures, attitudes and world view assist the therapist in examining the service user and in recognising and understanding the key signs. In the case of psychoanalysis, the trained ear of the therapist is constantly looking for meaningful clues that often only he or she is able to recognise. These clues and transparencies are frequently missed by the interpreter, who, rather than translating directly, naturally interprets meanings.

The interpreting agency

Matching the right interpreter to the right occasion by taking into account all the issues raised above is the job of an interpreting agency. In addition, the agency has a host of other factors to contend with, not least of which is the problem of supply and demand. This takes place alongside the usual daily routine of business management including recruitment, training and accounting (invoicing, credit control and payroll) together with data and general office management. The task, if the agency is to be successful, is to be able to balance this equation against a background of unknown and unpredictable fluctuations.

To be able to meet the demands of the market place the provision of interpreting services requires in-depth market analysis. It is vital to establish how much need there exists for such a service. However, it is perhaps even more important to establish from the outset how such needs are funded. The first issue to recognise is that the decision makers in buying interpreting services are not necessarily the users of the service. They are the bureaucrats at managerial level with limited understanding of community interpreting. Of course the most effective managers are the ones who consult regularly with their staff, but do these organisations or individuals believe in the effectiveness and importance of the service? Furthermore, if the users are either obliged by law to appreciate the provision, or are to be educated to do so, can their raised expectations be met realistically?

It is worthwhile to examine the level of interpreting needed in a community, with all its peculiar difficulties. It may be that the statistics and figures obtained cannot be taken for granted or do not lead to concrete conclusions. Nevertheless the exercise is the first step to understanding and appreciating the industry, and in particular the community and the needs of its members. A considerable amount of work has been undertaken in the past in ethnic monitoring and in language surveys using data from population censuses and other social surveys. These statistics play an important role in determining the level of need. Accurate conclusions and assessment are, however, extremely difficult to reach.

Various factors influence the final outcome of such research. For example, the interpreting requirements of a small but newly arrived refugee group far exceed the needs of a large but long established immigrant population. In the early to mid-90s, whilst a number of prominent academic institutions and community interpreting organisations were engaged in their valuable work of training interpreters from mainly Asian backgrounds, London was hungry for bilingual Somalis. This was due to the sudden influx of Somali refugees into the UK at the time. It starkly illustrates the weakness of ethnic monitoring in general and the unpredictable nature of the need for interpreters of different languages in particular.

Another factor in the level of usage of the services by non-English speaking groups is how effectively the services are publicised, especially in and for minority languages.

A further factor which leads to an increase in the need for interpreting services is a general lack of, or exhaustion of, resources. Reductions in the level of welfare benefits, sudden influxes of refugee groups nationally or locally, administrative crises in any public sector department, and so on can easily lead, either on a national or local level, to the withdrawal of services and benefits. This in turn leads to more stringent assessment interviews, calling inevitably for longer interpreting sessions. It takes less time, energy and planning to say 'yes' to a service user than to say 'no'. When a department is unable to supply the need, not only does the reason for rejection have to be explained and justified, but on most occasions alternative routes must also be recommended. Of course alternative routes mean more interviews and an increased need for interpreters.

However there can be bizarre consequences of using interpreters. For instance on some occasions the cost of interpreting may even exceed the cost of fulfilling the service user's need in the first place. I recall an occasion when an applicant who had recently been housed paid a visit to the Benefits Agency to ask for a crisis loan, in order to buy bedding at a cost of £30. The Benefits Agency used an interpreting agency to speak to the person on the telephone. The conversation took a long time. The applicant's request for £30 was turned down. The bill for the telephone interpreter was £63.

Telephone interpreting, the simple process of connecting an interpreter via a telephone line to the interview room, is an important development in the world of community interpreting and it is becoming an increasingly important demand on interpreting agencies. Amongst its major advantages is that there are no travel costs and the organisers of the service have full control over when the interpreter actually attends the interview. The disadvantages speak for themselves. Telephone interpreting may be immediate, but it is always rushed. There is no time for the preliminary warm-up period desirable when sensitive issues are to be discussed. The important element of body language is missing from the conversation and it lacks a host of other significant elements that contribute to a successful interview. It is at times as inappropriate as making a proposal of marriage over the phone.

The telephone service, in the field of mental health, is best used for making appointments for future meetings or, in an emergency only, to assess immediate need. In general it is most successful if used to pass on simple messages only. It is worth noting that the convenience of having an interpreter immediately available has made this form of interpreting increasingly popular.

Let us now turn our attention to the supply side of the equation and to the availability of interpreters to meet demand. Ideally the most appropriate interpreter will be supplied for each assignment. It is therefore of primary importance that interpreters receive the necessary training. There are a number of institutions and local bodies that provide community interpreting courses at different levels of proficiency. In addition many interpreting agencies conduct in-house training for the interpreters registered with the organisation. To have been trained, as with any other profession, is considered either a necessary criterion, or at least a major bonus when it comes to recruitment.

The first problem with training requirements is that employers tend to be very stringent in their selection of interpreters of more common languages where the supply is plentiful, and very flexible with interpreters of more exotic languages. Often with uncommon languages there is no choice but to use the available interpreters irrespective of their level of training.

The second problem is that trained interpreters are by nature more career oriented, and for that reason may only be in the industry temporarily before going on to a more secure position. This of course means that a constant supply of fresh interpreters must be recruited and resources allocated to training them.

Finally it must be mentioned that it is impossible, or at least unethical, to force or even encourage individuals to receive time-consuming training for a profession that will not offer them sufficient work and an adequate living. This is unfortunately the reality with all less common languages where the need for an interpreter is insufficient to guarantee any form of part-time or even sessional employment.

This is perhaps the biggest obstacle to community interpreting evolving into a profession because no agency can be sure of the level of demand for interpreters in a given language. Of course there are rare examples of short-term contracts given to interpreters by some organisations, but this can hardly provide the security required to pursue a profession. Enhancement of their own skills, additional training, or even a university degree do not in any way promise a future in the field. It is therefore no surprise that most interpreters use the job as a stepping stone to other more secure professions. In a recent survey conducted among 200 community interpreters working for one agency, only 4.5 per cent said that they look on their work as a career and wish to continue in the industry. Most view interpreting as a way to pay the bills while planning to pursue other careers or education in the future.

On a more optimistic note, many interpreters find suitable professions through their interpreting work. I know of a number of examples where part-time interpreters have become social workers, refugee workers and counsellors, though others do find their permanent niche in a variety of different professions.

A morning at the agency

As I unlock the office door early on Monday morning I can hear the phone ringing in the interpreting department. It could be an urgent booking, I had better rush! 'More haste, less speed,' I tell myself as I fumble with the lock. It finally opens; I am inside and half-way across the room when I realise there is a another loud noise welcoming me to work with its demand for instant attention. Of course! I've forgotten the security alarm. I rush back in the opposite direction, find the alarm panel, enter the code and to my relief the siren is stilled, giving prominence once again to the insistent call of the telephone. One more sprint and I might just make it. Unfortunately my last stride is in vain: as my hand touches the receiver the ringing stops. I collapse onto the nearest chair and quickly review all the people who may have been desperate enough to ring so early. Could it be one of them? Will they ring again? Or will I hear too late: 'I phoned to warn you, but there was no answer.'

It really is too early for such a rush of adrenalin, particularly as I like to be able to savour the early morning calm of the office as a chance to reflect and take stock. The alarm and phone are still ringing in my ears, but this gradually gives way to the hubbub of activity as my colleagues start arriving one by one and I join in the early morning coffee ritual. People are talking, phones start ringing and the familiar rush of the office builds up as the day gets into full swing.

It is going to be another busy day. We have dozens of people booked on assignments. The monthly wages were paid last week, so we are bound to get some queries today. I have already taken several calls from interpreters needing street directions, plus a booking for a language I have never heard of. That will require careful research in the language database. The first phone call to one of my colleagues was from an Arabic interpreter calling in sick and cancelling an 11.00 a.m. assignment in east London. My colleague has already called the service user, more out of courtesy than caution, as Arabic bookings are not difficult to fill even at such short notice. Had the service user had special gender or dialect requests it might have been a different matter. The same interpreter has an appointment for tomorrow as well. I wonder if he is going to be able to make it. We will have to give him a call later to make sure he is all right. The list of memos and reminders on my desk is already half a page long and it is still only 9.30 a.m.

Another colleague has just finished opening the post and as head of the section, a sheaf of letters is passed to me. I am afraid there is a written complaint about an interpreter on a home visit. Our interpreter was asked to meet a health visitor at the service user's home. Arriving a few minutes early she was invited by the service user to wait inside her house. By the time the health visitor arrived the interpreter and the service user were busy drinking tea and chatting about their homeland. The letter explains that the interpreter and the health visitor should have arrived together. As it was, it was more difficult for them to work as a team and, more importantly, to appear to the service user to be a team. The health visitor claims that this could also have jeopardised the interpreter's impartiality. I will have to discuss the issues with both parties in order to prevent similar difficulties in the future. But even despite our best efforts I remember we have already had this problem before. On one occasion the interpreter claimed that she felt safer indoors. She also explained that she saw it as part of her brief to gain the service user's trust to ensure a successful interview. To have refused a compatriot's invitation into her home would have been to cause offence. I am sure there is a policy statement or a guideline on this issue in our material somewhere, but as with all matters relating to society and people, there is no absolutely correct answer. In the end it really all depends on the circumstances.

My thoughts are interrupted by the call of the telephone again:

'Hello, interpreting department, how may I help you?'
'Good morning. We have a service user from Ethiopia, do you have anyone who speaks Ethiopian?'
'You mean Amharic. Yes?'
'Well I don't know. All I know is that he comes from Ethiopia. Maybe I can ask him. What did you say the language was?'
'Amharic!'
'Ah yes, if you can hold a few moments I will find out.'

It is always difficult in these circumstances. There can be so many languages spoken in a single country, yet so many different countries where the same language is spoken. It is always a stimulating challenge trying to advise service users on the interpreter they need, but if we get it wrong we have to take the blame. Unfortunately it is not as simple as looking it up on a list as there are often so many political issues to take into account. And as political events unfold, so realities change. Just because an interpreter speaks the same language as the interviewee, this does not itself provide the solution. A recent example is the status of Serbian and Croatian. Even though these are essentially the same language, few Croatians would admit that they understand a Serb or agree to have a Serb interpreter. The problem gets more complicated when . . .

'Hello, are you still there?'
'Yes I am.'
'My service user shook his head to Amharic. What else could he speak?'
'Maybe your service user is from Eritrea, in which case he would speak Tigrinya.'
'No I know he is from Ethiopia.'
'Yes but Eritrea was a part of Ethiopia up until a few years ago before they gained their independence. Amharic was the

national language and from what I know everyone had to learn Amharic at school. But not everyone from what today is Eritrea necessarily speaks Amharic.'

'So you reckon Tigrinya, right? How do you spell that?'

I wish all the calls were as easy to solve.

Time sheets, time sheets and more time sheets. In the post, by fax, they are piling up on my desk and they all need to be checked and passed to the accounts department for invoicing and payment. As I walk in they are all involved in a serious discussion.

'What is happening?' I ask.

'Nothing special,' says one of my colleagues. 'Just another letter from an interpreter concerned about the deductions of tax and National Insurance.'

'That is at least the third one this month,' adds another.

'What is their point this time?' I ask.

He lifts the letter closer to his eyes and, as if looking for something that he knows is not there, he zooms in and says, 'Nothing new, same old thing. He says that when he works for himself on interpreting assignments in court or for solicitors or hospitals, no tax is deducted, but when he works for the agency, he is taxed.'

I seek the warm sanctuary of the kettle again. I have been involved in numerous similar conversations about tax, National Insurance and entitlement to benefits in relation to community interpreting. Yes, we have spoken about it, we have attended conferences on it, read guidelines and whole books on it, but it seems to be one of those issues that is not tackled comprehensively and for which no one can offer an appropriate solution. Community interpreting work takes place under so many different circumstances involving the health service, other public sector agencies and the legal system. All these organisations have their own systems of payment. First, the law is open to interpretation on whether interpreters are self-employed or should be taxed at source. Second, if an organisation employs an interpreter on an ad-hoc basis only, it is unlikely that they will find it practical to get involved with the PAYE system. The result is that in practice interpreters are responsible for their own tax affairs on some jobs for some organisations, but are taxed on others.

As far as the Benefits Agency is concerned the rules show little tolerance or allow little flexibility for sessional workers who work irregular hours on moderate salaries, and who may be busy today, but have no work for weeks at a time. This is especially true with the more uncommon languages where work comes one's way very sporadically. I know of a number of occasions when interpreters have declined work or have suggested doing the work on a voluntary basis because it did not make financial sense to accept the job.

The fact is that community interpreting is an odd profession. In many senses it is even wrong to consider it a profession at all. Putting aside other forms of interpreting, for example interpreting for international conferences in the political arena or for commercial organisations, an interpreter has less security, less control, and, most importantly, less recognition than most other freelance workers. Very few community interpreters are paid a regular salary, but that is still on a temporary contract, and in general interpreters are sessional workers with few or no rights at all. They are never guaranteed work by any organisation. This is simply because no organisation can be sure of the need for interpreters in a given language. There may be occasions when, due to the influx of certain ethnic minority groups, a particular language enjoys a brief surge of demand and new interpreters are recruited in that language. But my experience is that if there are any promises of employment they are almost certainly short-term and at most, subject to requirements.

I return to my desk to find more time sheets have appeared. One has a complaint attached to it – about our charge for travelling time. We charge and pay for the time it takes the interpreter to travel to and from the venue. A disgruntled solicitor has written:

> My colleagues and I commute between our places of residence and work on a daily basis, but we do not charge our service users for this. Our charges for our services are based solely on the time spent on our service users. I therefore fail to comprehend, and more importantly to legitimise in my mind, the fees your company is imposing for the time spent by your employees travelling.

We have had this a number of times too. The point is, when a solicitor, social worker, or for that matter anyone in full time employment leaves home in the morning, they are guaranteed work and therefore payment for the duration of the day. Community interpreting bookings, on the other hand, are rarely for more than a few hours. If an interpreter is allocated a 1-hour assignment even within the boundaries of London, he or she must set aside at least half a day for that assignment when travelling time is taken into account. For the same reason it is very rare that we can give an interpreter more than two assignments in a day because of the problem of travelling between venues. It would be completely unfair only to pay an interpreter for 2 hours of work that has in effect taken the whole day to accomplish.

As I am deep in my thoughts, my phone starts ringing again. A doctor wants to book a female Cantonese interpreter for an assessment. We actually have a whole week's notice which makes it easier to organise. I quickly put the information into the computer and start calling our interpreters to see who is available. But I am interrupted by an incoming call bringing another problem:

'Hello, we have one of your interpreters with us.'

'Yes, how can I help?'

'Well we asked for an Albanian interpreter and you have sent us someone from . . . uh . . . somewhere else.'

'Is our interpreter from Kosovo?' I ask.

'Yes that's it. Kosovo. Our service user says he does not want to be interviewed with this interpreter,' says the caller.

'Is there a language problem?' I ask, thinking immediately that the difficulty probably lies elsewhere.

'I don't know. Why? This is your mistake isn't it? I didn't ask for Kosovan,' says the caller, beginning to raise his voice.

'Yes I know, but they speak the same language. They shouldn't have any problems communicating,' I reply reassuringly. 'Did you specifically ask for someone from Albania?'

'It is not my job to know who speaks what language. As far as I am concerned I have asked you for an Albanian interpreter and you confirmed you could send me an Albanian interpreter. Your interpreter is not from Albania.'

'But you see, when you asked for an Albanian interpreter you meant the language not the country. The overwhelming majority of Albanian speakers in this country are from Kosovo, not Albania.'

'Well if my service user refuses to work with your interpreter then there must be something wrong. I don't know . . .'

'Could we perhaps use the interpreter to arrange another interview?'
'I don't know, let me find out. I will call you back.' He hangs up.

As I hang up my phone I mutter to myself. 'These areas of political or religious difference can be as unpredictable as they are difficult to solve.'

'Are you still with us? Wake up' says my colleague jokingly from the next desk. 'I'm here. I was just thinking how many things can go wrong,' I reply.
'I know. You were talking to yourself again. What was this one about? Politics, religion, accent, dialect, gender or . . .?'
'You sound as if you're reading from a text book.'
'I went on a course a few weeks ago about interpreting and all the issues involved. You know, the fact that some of it goes according to plan without any hassles is a miracle.'
'You don't need to tell me that.'
'The course leader was fascinating. He started by talking about how we have been born and brought up constantly forming opinions about anything and everything around us. He said we do this as naturally and as unconsciously as we breathe. It is second nature to us. Yet interpreters, since they play a central role in conversations dealing with some of the most intimate details of people's lives, have to remain completely detached and uninvolved. They are supposed to look interested in order to gain everyone's trust, but everything they hear should have absolutely no impact at all. How can anyone do that?'
'Well if you learn it professionally you get used to it.'
'OK, maybe in a commercial atmosphere or even in legal cases you can distance yourself, but when you are working with the community and are so involved with everyone's life, it's impossible. Even a judge and jury who are supposed to be impartial are expected to form an opinion and reach a verdict, but an interpreter's job is to never allow herself to even think about exactly what is happening.'

I can see her point and we prepare to embark on another fruitful discussion on community interpreting, but as usual her phone starts ringing and another highly stimulating subject gives way to the advent of practicality and the arrangements for another booking. My own immediate task is a fax that has just arrived on my desk. It is from a doctor in a local hospital asking for an interpreter in Swahili with experience in interpreting for mental health service users. Before calling the service user I continue reading the requirements. Unfortunately as I read on, the order gets increasingly challenging. The request is for a female Swahili speaker from Kenya who specialises in mental health and who has worked with families in the past. It also specifies that her English must be at a level suitable for her to attend mental health tribunals. The last requirement is that she should be free for the next three Tuesdays, although no guarantee can be given that the work will be available since the meetings are to be confirmed later after consultation with several hospital staff and doctors. Before calling the doctor I take a quick look at our database. We have twenty-one Swahili interpreters free on the day of the first appointment. Only ten are from Kenya, of which three are female. Of these one is geographically close enough to the hospital. She does not specialise in mental health and is only available at the weekend due to full time employment.

I need to speak directly to the doctor in charge to establish, and hopefully negotiate, the priorities. Unfortunately the requirements for bookings are often too specific and, depending on the language, we may be unable to supply the exact interpreter required. On these occasions we put almost as much effort into clarifying the situation with the service user as we put into selecting the most appropriate interpreter. It is better to be realistic and share the bad news with our service users in advance. Sadly, if we are unable to fulfil the request exactly, there are few alternatives for them but to compromise on some aspects of their requirement and accept the most appropriate interpreter available.

It is almost time for lunch and I turn to warn my colleague that I am leaving my desk for a short while. Unfortunately she is busy on a phone call. Maybe I will wait for a few minutes until she has finished. Then my own phone rings again.

'Hello, how can I help you?'
'Hello, could I speak to the lady in the interpreting department please?'
'I'm afraid she is on the phone. Can I help you?'

'We booked an interpreter for an ante-natal emergency this morning. The lady I spoke to was very helpful and the interpreter arrived very quickly.'

'I'm very pleased we could help.'

'I sounded so desperate this morning and couldn't talk much. Anyway, I am just calling to say thank you to her and to let her know how good the interpreter was. And she will want to know it was a boy. Eight pounds and five ounces.'

'I'll pass the news onto her. She will be delighted. Thank you so much for calling.'

'We have told the mother to make sure her son applies to your agency as soon as he starts talking.'

'We will make sure we send him an application form!'

It is all well worth it in the end and it is with a sense of high elation that we set off for a well-earned lunch.

Chapter 6

An interpreter's perspective

Minoo Razban

Introduction

In a multicultural society that consists of people who have recently migrated to Britain, and for whom English will be a second language, being able to negotiate basic life transactions will be fraught with difficulties due to the absence of the English language. Being able to learn English may provide a medium to long-term solution, but in the immediacy of having to get health or other practical needs met an interpreter may provide the only lifeline. As new communities have migrated to Britain, so the need for interpreters has increased. However, in being able to find the right fit between the interpreter and a service user, due consideration has to be given to matching for dialect, religion, language, culture, country of origin, and ethnicity to mention a few variables. Interpreters from the same country may not share the same dialect or ethnicity for example.

The state of the problem

Most of us talk to friends or family when faced with difficulties or problems, but there may be times when this does not feel appropriate and we may want to talk with an outsider or professional. Talking with people we know well may actually make the problem worse. There are likely to be cultural taboos that make it difficult to talk about certain types of difficulties with family members or professional helpers, such as those related to mental health. Mental health carries a stigma in most communities, and may be associated with increased anxiety for the individual or their family when such problems are acknowledged. The situation may intensify and

become more distressing as an individual finds it increasingly difficult to communicate their distress to others, especially when not
having the language of the host community by which to share this
distress with others. An interpreter will play an invaluable role in
helping the person seeking professional help for their mental health
needs. It is at this point that the interpreter's role becomes vital.
The interpreter has to gain the trust of the professional and the
service user, and has to ensure accurate translation, in order to
create the foundation from which the therapeutic work may begin.
The interpreter may also need to act as a broker for the professional, and provide the service user with an understanding of the
service context, as this may be unfamiliar to the service user. It is
important to ensure that all the parties, who are involved in the
process of either receiving or providing a therapeutic intervention,
are properly briefed and know what to expect from each other.

Criteria for good interpreting

The interpreter is central to the process of good communication,
and it is therefore important that the role of the interpreter is
clearly defined, and that it falls within the level of skill and experience of the interpreter. The types of skills needed by an interpreter
are given below:

- Fluency in the languages being used by the professional and
  the service user, and a good knowledge of any dialects being
  used within a given language, if required.
- Having relevant medical or psychological knowledge, and
  ability to communicate the essence of such information across
  the two languages involved.
- Sensitivity towards the service user and his or her mental health
  needs, and respective family members of the service user.
- Confidentiality applies for all types of interpreting, but in
  mental health it is especially important because of the stigma
  attached to mental illness.
- Experience and training within the mental health field.

Techniques of interpreting

There needs to be a good level of co-operation between the
interpreter and the clinician if the interpreter is going to be able to

carry out the task of interpreting well. The clinician has to communicate in a coherent, concise and precise manner to make the job of translation easier for the interpreter. The following broad 'rules of thumb' go a long way to making the job of the interpreter easier:

- Translating after a person has finished speaking is normally how the interpreter works. However, simultaneous interpreting can also be very useful (e.g. when the professional is interviewing a family with an interpreter).
- Any disagreement about the way of interpreting, or any cultural question from the interpreter, should not take place in front of the service user. This issue makes the pre-session briefing or a brief break for discussion very important. For example, professionals sometimes misinterpret the interpreter's need to repeat a question, or have a longer conversation with the service user in order to gain better clarity or understanding of the service user's difficulties, as taking over the work. The mistrust sensed by the interpreter, as well as the service user, can make all the parties concerned feel uncomfortable.
- The clinician should bear in mind that he should not talk continuously for more than two or at most three minutes. It is impractical and impossible for the interpreter to memorise the clinician's words accurately when the clinician talks for more than two or three minutes. The amount of spoken information that the clinician generates is best kept brief, so that the interpreter can render an accurate and meaningful translation to the service user. Ideally, the interpretation should be carried out word for word in order to convey the message of the clinician sincerely and accurately, but in order to preserve the meaning of the communication the interpreter may need to take longer.

Briefing

All individuals, who are involved in a therapy session, including the clinician, the service user and the interpreter, should develop an accurate understanding of the service user's difficulties. This is particularly important for the interpreter, as he or she has a pivotal role in rendering an accurate understanding of the service user's difficulties to the clinician. Therefore, it is vital that the interpreter is sufficiently trained and has the right level of experience in being able to carry out mental health work, as stated earlier.

In general, a good working relationship should be established between all the parties concerned (i.e. the service user–interpreter, interpreter–clinician and the clinician–service user), in order to ensure that the communication between the clinician and the service user is maximised. The latter can be enhanced through having briefing sessions between the interpreter and the clinician, during the course of the therapy.

For example, a 10- to 15-minute pre-session briefing before the first interview is helpful in order to have a better understanding of respective roles in the work, and to discuss the following types of issues:

- The clinician briefs the interpreter about the situation and discusses the possible course of the first session. This should include the way that the clinician wishes the interpreter to work.
- The clinician learns and practices the accurate pronunciation of the service user's name to ensure that the name of the service user will be pronounced correctly. A mispronunciation of the name can create a barrier between the service user and the clinician, and the service user may feel the clinician has not spent sufficient time preparing beforehand.
- It is usually valuable to negotiate beforehand the possibility of having a discussion outside of the room between the interpreter and the clinician if difficulties are being identified in their working relationship within the room. The two may need time to discuss issues that may be causing distress to the service user (e.g. the service user is becoming uncomfortable with the line of questioning).

It is helpful for the clinician to ensure that the service user and the interpreter are kept abreast of the line of enquiry or treatment approach being used. Familiarity and predictability can help to alleviate unnecessary anxiety and stress that a service user or interpreter is faced with in an unfamiliar mental health context. The clinician will also need to develop an awareness of and be able to deal with practical issues that may be brought by the service user in the context of a mental health consultation, such as housing problems. The clinician will need to be sensitive to how such factors may be impacting on the service user's mental health, and to develop ways in which they may be able to support the service user with their practical needs if the clinician feels unable to do this in the context of providing therapy. At other times, providing direct support to the service user (e.g. letter of support to the housing department) may go a long way towards promoting the therapeutic engagement and positive clinical outcome.

Tension in the work

Interpreters often have to straddle the tensions created in mental health work, and have to strike a delicate balance between remaining impartial or neutral, whilst knowing when their own views and reactions may need to become more explicit if the therapeutic work is not going to be jeopardised. Clarifying points of uncertainty or the way a clinician prefers to work before seeing the service user can help the interpreter to become more familiar with the service context. It also helps with building up the working relationship and trust between the interpreter and the clinician.

Service users may repeat information that they have given in the course of the interview, and the interpreter has to understand why the service user is finding it necessary to provide the information again. The interpreter should also bear in mind that the meaning behind the service user's words not only describes his mental problems, but it is also a reflection of his mental state. Therefore, a sincere interpretation of the service user is a vital part of the therapy as this helps the clinician to diagnose the service user's problem by understanding the service user's situation correctly. It is also extremely important that the interpreter speaks in the first person.

The best compliment that I have ever had was when I had been asked to interpret for a child. After the session, the clinician told me that for the first time they had not felt the presence of the interpreter in the room, and that it had felt as if they had talked directly with the child.

Impartiality

A while ago, I met a service user, for whom I used to interpret at the same clinic. Another interpreter had been called to interpret for the service user's last assessment appointment. The service user's understanding of English was good, but his spoken English was limited. The service user told me:

> I knew exactly what I was saying and it should not have been the interpreter's business, nor should it have mattered to the interpreter, if the interpreter thought that what I was saying was wrong or inappropriate. The interpreter should have interpreted in such a way that I would have said, had I been able to speak English myself. The interpreter had summarised my sentences rather than interpreting my sentences as they had been spoken. The interpreter should have said what I had asked them to say.

The service user held the belief that he would not have been sectioned, had the interpreter carried out the translation sincerely and without any deviations from his original words.

The above situation is an example of the types of problems that can occur within the interpreter–service user working relationship. A balance has to be struck between providing verbatim translation and summary translation, whilst still conveying accurately what the service user is communicating. Interpreters must bear in mind that it is not their job to decide what would be helpful and advantageous for the service user. The only real assistance and help to the service users is to convey their words as they have said, without being biased and leaving the diagnosis and the treatment to the clinician.

Continuity and trust

It is usually better to have the same interpreter present through a piece of work with the service user, as this is likely to facilitate trust and provide continuity. Having the same interpreter will also increase the efficacy of the work. The same interpreter can hold the service user's story about their problem and provide containment through a piece of work; both of which are lost when a service user has to relate to different interpreters at each appointment with the clinician. In order to convey the non-verbal and verbal emotional information, it can sometimes be helpful for the interpreter to match the tone and intonation being expressed by the service user. This may be of particular importance in maintaining the therapeutic alliance with a service user who is expressing very painful information about him or her self. The interpreter will also have to manage their reactions to the material particularly when this may be causing embarrassment or resonating with the interpreter. With difficult clinical material such as sexual problems an interpreter may laugh out of embarrassment, but this will jeopardise the work and relationship with the service user. Again, briefing and debriefing sessions can go some way towards anticipating the possible areas of difficulty that may arise for the interpreter, and thereby create the opportunity of being able to discuss the issues before they have a negative impact on the work.

Concluding remarks

This chapter has been based on the author's personal experiences of working as an interpreter. The working relationships between the interpreter and the service user, and the interpreter and the clinician were thought about, and some of the problems that arise in these were discussed. However, this area of work is complex, and it needs further research and clinical thinking to be carried out. There is also a need for the work to be discussed and shared between interpreters and clinicians through joint teaching and information sharing through seminars and conferences. Guidelines for good practice in this area of work need to be developed and continually refined as this area of work develops in its own right.

Continuity between the clinician and the interpreter is also important in strengthening their working alliance, and again the more time they build in for briefing and debriefing, the better their working relationship will become. Containment and trust are also lost when the service user is faced with having to see different interpreters in subsequent appointments about the same problem. Interpreters have to build up trust with the service user and the clinician. Interpreters need to maintain a sensitive and sympathetic manner with the service user.

Chapter 7

The role and experience of interpreters

Emily Granger and Martyn Baker

Introduction

Clients in many settings are eager for culturally compatible professional practitioners[1] (e.g. Hillier et al, 1994). However, training sufficient ethnic minority professionals to match the ethnic profile of service users in the UK is patently impracticable under current training constraints, which fall lamentably short of this ideal – Boyle et al (1993), for example, have highlighted the difficulty of recruiting sufficient numbers of psychology graduates from ethnic minorities to clinical psychology training. With respect to those who do not sufficiently understand or speak English, the use of interpreting services is undoubtedly simpler, more practical and more economical. This chapter investigates the interpreters' experience in their work with human service professionals like social workers, lawyers, immigration staff, and medical staff, where some specific technical knowledge is required of the interpreter, but where equally importantly the interpreter will also be acting as a 'cultural broker' (Kaufert and Koolage, 1984).

Guidelines for using the services of interpreters in these sorts of situations do exist (Saunders and Broune, 1992; Shackman 1984). The literature informing such guidance tends to comprise discussion papers, often based upon anecdotal evidence, very often from medical settings, and almost exclusively from the viewpoint of the client, and of the practitioner.

---

[1] Throughout the chapter, professional service providers are referred to as 'practitioners', service users speaking only non-English languages are referred to as 'clients', and those providing interpreting services are referred to as 'interpreters'.

From the clients' perspective, the use of interpreters is reported to give a better:

sense of professional attention (Faust and Drickey, 1986)
sense of being understood (Kline et al, 1980)
return rate following initial assessment (Hillier et al, 1994)
sense of client/practitioner compatibility (Cox, 1977)

but may increase the risk of various problems:

various unhelpful coalitions –
   interpreter and practitioner versus client (Hillier et al, 1994)
   interpreter and client versus practitioner (Tribe, 1991)
   interpreter and one client versus practitioner and another client
      (Freed, 1988)

unhelpful intrusion of various negative emotional states in the
client –
   insulted because using the services of an interpreter implies client
      cannot speak majority language well enough (Harvey, 1984)
   belittled (Stansfield, 1981)
   inhibited by culturally inappropriate age, sex or social class of
      interpreter (Raval, 1996)

by content discussed –
   embarrassment (e.g. sexual matters; Cox, 1977)
   shame (e.g. issues of maternity; Owan, 1985)
   horror (e.g. political refugees; Tribe, 1991)

by suspicion of interpreter (Roe and Roe, 1991)

From the practitioners' perspective, the use of an interpreter is reported to give a:

generally positive reaction to the use of interpreting services
   (Raval, 1996)
increased respect for interpreters if they are trained (Raval, 1996)

but the practitioner may feel:

greater detachment from situation (Kline, Adrian and Spevak,
   1980; Raval, 1996)

threatened by a third party (the interpreter) observing their professional work (Raval, 1996)

frustrated –
- especially where *language* is the key professional tool (Raval, 1996)
- at the delay between understanding the non-verbal and the verbal communication (Roy, 1992)

hostile if the interpreter is thought to go beyond mere translation service (Kaufert and Koolage, 1984) and various resultant power struggles emerge (Good and Good, 1981; Tribe, 1991; Raval, 1996)

From the interpreters' perspective, Harvey (1984) reported they may become the object of the practitioner's defence mechanisms e.g. of displacement of feelings of decreased power; and Tribe (1991) noted interpreters working with political refugees and victims of torture may over-identify with the clients' accounts. Raval (1996) reports single case detail of the interpreter involved in his study. These apart, we have not uncovered other references to research reports from the perspective of the interpreters themselves.

Despite the fact that the 'voice' of interpreters is by and large missing from the literature, a string of recommendations exist within it, expressing a 'voice' drawn from practitioners and clients. These amount almost to a 'good practice' guide when using interpreters in professional situations (see Chapter 3 in this book). The clear need is that the experience of interpreters themselves should be investigated, and that any guidelines for practice should also be informed by what they say.

Thus the research reported here was planned to be an empirical study, deliberately targeting interpreters themselves to ask them about their work experience. In order to reach a large number of participants, it was decided to contact interpreters working over a variety of service agencies, using relevant issues highlighted in the available literature to develop the questionnaire.

The interpreters' experiences

The interpreters' experiences described in the sections that follow are based on the empirical study carried out by Granger (1996), and specific details of the methodology and research analysis can be found there. The key findings from 64 returned questionnaires from the 300 sent out to interpreters are summarised below. The quantitative information from the questionnaires was analysed using statistical analysis, details of which are given in Granger (1996).

Demographic characteristics of the participants are given in Table 7.1. There were equal proportions of females and males, and twice as many older as younger. Most spoke between two and four languages fluently. Although over half had received no formal training as interpreters, the participants as a whole were academically highly educated, and the professional qualifications they reported included those in nursing, medicine, law, journalism, engineering and architecture. Their continuing motivation for training was reflected in the high proportion currently working towards further qualification.

Two-thirds had been employed as interpreters for a period of 5 years or less. Their work fell between 'casual' and 'freelance', involving being 'on call' for the employing organisation. About two-thirds currently obtained work as interpreters for only 4 or less hours per week, with a further third working up to 16 hours per week. Only a handful reported more than 16 hours. Many participants were engaged in multiple tasks – for instance, over 40 per cent were simultaneously involved in further education and professional training. The interpreting work was spread across multiple agencies – Local Authority social services, legal services, refugee services and health services were most often cited. Since the location of such services is not centralised, participants had to travel to multiple worksites.

Participants' experience of the work situation

As shown in Table 7.2, participants overwhelmingly agreed their role to be that of language translators. Other aspects received considerably less endorsement, though cultural brokerage, explaining technical terms, rapport building, and client advocacy were the main ones acknowledged. The role expectations they felt clients and practitioners had for them were substantially similarly endorsed; though they indicated the function of 'cultural broker' was less expected of them than they themselves recognised it to be an important part of the work. The vast majority felt their role did

Table 7.1   Demographic characteristics of participants (*N* = 64)

Sex:
Female	53%
Male	47%

Age:
18–35 years	36%
36+ years	64%

Number of languages spoken fluently:
2	34%
3	31%
4	21%
5	8%
6+	6%

Education and training:
Specifically as interpreter
Formally trained	19%
Short course	26%
None	55%

Professional qualifications
Professionally trained	30%
Not so trained	70%

Level of academic qualifications
School examinations only	22%
Further education certificate	8%
Undergraduate degree	42%
Postgraduate qualification	28%

Currently undergoing further qualification
Yes	41%
No	59%

Work experience as interpreter:
Years worked as interpreter
5 years or less	66%
Over 5 years	34%

Current hours per week
4 hours or less	61%
Between 5 and 16 hours	31%
More than 16 hours	8%

Work settings:
Social services	83%
Legal services	80%
Refugee services	66%
Medical health services	50%
Mental health services	31%
Commercial services	16%

Table 7.2   Details of how participants (*N* = 64) felt about the work situation

Work situation	Feelings of participants (N = 64)	
Aspects of the role of the interpreter:	*Self-perceived*	Perceived expectations (by client and practitioner)
Language translator	95%	89%
Explain cultural factors to practitioner	53%	43%
Explain technical terms to client	51%	56%
Build rapport between practitioner and client	48%	50%
Client advocate	44%	39%
Persuade client to comply with practitioner's wishes	17%	21%
Befriend client	12%	18%

Changes in role when working with client from another culture to own:	
No change	76%
Role *would* change because –	
know less about client's circumstances	14%
know less about political factors	14%
know less about client's culture	12%
know less about social factors	12%
less well able to establish rapport with client	10%

Biasing effect upon interview content, due solely to the presence of an interpreter:	*More likely to be talked about*	*Less likely*
Social issues	84%	6%
Political issues	73%	10%
Legal issues	73%	6%
Issues that confuse the client	70%	12%
Family issues	64%	18%
Cultural issues	59%	14%
Marital issues	51%	32%
Psychological issues	32%	26%
Sexual issues	32%	60%

Difficulties experienced working as an interpreter:	
Not having enough knowledge of client's culture	37%
Not having enough time to build rapport	32%
Not having technical terms explained	29%

continues overleaf

Table 7.2   (continued)

Not knowing the purpose of the interview	28%
Not having time to explain cultural factors	26%
Not being treated with respect by the practitioner	21%
Not having time to explain technicalities	21%
Difficulty in translating technical terms	20%
Not feeling comfortable with the nature of the material discussed	12%
Not being treated with respect by the client	12%
Not knowing enough about the client's circumstances	9%
Not feeling comfortable about the sex of the practitioner	6%
Not feeling comfortable about the sex of the client	4%
Possible helps towards resolving the difficulties:	
Pre- and post-interview meetings with practitioner	53%
Being informed about the purpose of the interview	42%
Practitioner being trained to work with an interpreter	34%
Being trained in technical terms	31%
More time allocated for interviews	29%
Receiving formal training and professional status	28%
Being treated with greater respect	26%
Being informed about client's culture before the interview	21%
Interpreters being matched with client (appropriate age, sex, culture)	6%

not alter between situations where they shared the client's language *and* cultural background, and situations where *only* the language was shared.

Where interviews involved an interpreter being present, certain topics were identified by participants as being more facilitated than hindered by their presence (social issues, political issues, legal issues, issues which confused the client, family issues and cultural issues). Perhaps more importantly, however, practitioner–client discussion of two topics was viewed by some as being facilitated and by others as being hindered by their presence (marital issues and psychological issues); and all reported discussion of sexual issues as being hindered by their presence.

The report of difficulties experienced in the interpreting situation indicates how little the 'guidance' listed on pp. 46–48 and pp. 61–64 of this book was experienced as being adhered to. Eight of the problem areas were endorsed by over 20 per cent of participants, including such basic things as not being informed of the purpose of an interview, and being allotted insufficient time to build rapport or explain cultural factors. One of the demands of working for

Table 7.3   Likert Scale section of Questionnaire – results rescaled
into three categories (N = 64)

	Categories		
Results	*High*	*Medium*	*Low*
1 Feel confident/competent in role:	86%	9%	5%
2 Satisfaction with interpreting work:	86%	8%	6%
3 Desire to change job:	34%	30%	36%
4 Tend to develop good rapport:			
With clients	74%	19%	7%
With practitioners	60%	28%	8%
5 Sense of work being valued:			
By clients	77%	19%	4%
By practitioners	57%	23%	20%
6 Need for formal training to work as/with interpreter:			
For interpreters	67%	25%	8%
For practitioners	50%	25%	25%

diverse services was evidenced by the fact that three of these
problem areas had to do with understanding and communicating
technicalities, which differ from agency to agency. The item most
participants indicated as a difficulty, was *not having enough
knowledge of the client's culture* (though curiously, *prior knowledge
of client's culture* figured comparatively low – eighth out of nine –
on the list of possible resolutions to the difficulties). Endorsement
of various resolutions of these work difficulties followed very much
the sort of 'good practice' indicators given on pp. 46–48 and pp.
61–64 of this book – except that hardly any participants suggested
that the culturally appropriate matching of interpreters for clients'
age and sex would be helpful.

As shown in Table 7.3, participants' very high job confidence
and job satisfaction ratings contrast curiously with the two-thirds
who expressed *high* or *medium* desire to change from working as an
interpreter, to some other occupation. Ratings of ability to establish rapport, and of the sense of being valued, show a considerably
more muted experience working with practitioners than with
clients. Finally, ratings of the need for formal training in working
in the interpreting situation did not reflect the 'good practice
recommendations' given in Chapter 3 – only two-thirds of the
participants felt this was highly needed for interpreters, and only
half felt it was so for practitioners.

Comparisons between different demographic groups

Older versus younger participants

Older participants were more likely to have worked as an interpreter for 5+ years. They were also more likely to have obtained a professional qualification, while younger participants were the ones more likely still to be studying for qualifications.

Female versus male participants

Men rated themselves higher in job confidence than women.

Education and training

Higher levels of *educational performance* were associated with greater job confidence (although educational level was *not* significantly related to job satisfaction). Lower levels were associated with a greater tendency to have worked as an interpreter for 5+ years, and to feeling that there was insufficient time allotted for interviews.

Having *professional qualifications* was associated with wanting to find alternative employment. It was also correlated with a differing sense of the role of the interpreter – such participants were less likely to see it as involving being the client's cultural advisor or befriender, as being part of their job to persuade the client to comply with the practitioner, or to discuss politics in the interview, and more likely to see it as part of their job to explain technical aspects of the particular service concerned. Professionally qualified participants were not likely to be currently engaged in further training. Those who were so engaged, had a greater desire to change their job than their qualified counterparts, and a greater tendency to report that practitioners treated them without respect. The greater the extent of *formal training as an interpreter*, the more likely participants were to have been working as an interpreter for 5+ years.

Length of service (5+ years versus 5 years or less)

In addition to those aspects already mentioned above, those who had worked for over 5 years as an interpreter were more likely to state they needed more time allowed for explaining technicalities to clients and cultural factors to practitioners, and for building appropriate rapport between the two. They were more likely to report experiencing disrespect from practitioners, and place higher value upon pre- and post-interview discussions. Ironically these more experienced interpreters were also significantly more likely to want to change their profession, and this was also the case for those few who worked over 16 hours per week as interpreters.

Summary of main quantitative results

- The work pattern was irregular, multi-location and multi-agency (one associated complication of this latter fact was the need to have sufficient specialist knowledge of the technicalities of several agencies).
- Participants reported high job confidence (and they were in fact generally highly qualified, or studying for further qualifications); however their work as interpreters co-exists with a substantial desire to find alternative employment.
- They reported high job satisfaction despite major hindrances to doing the job; their agreement with how these difficulties might be resolved follows fairly closely the 'guidelines' given in Chapter 3, except for the desirability of cultural matching.
- Being present as an interpreter may hinder the client's discussion of marital, psychological and especially sexual issues. In addition to being a translator, being an interpreter includes being cultural broker, technical explainer, rapport agent and advocate. The role is experienced as altering little with clients' differing cultural backgrounds.
- The demographic group significantly associated with most other factors was those who have worked as *interpreters for more than 5 years*. They tended to be older (36+ years); to have had formal training as interpreters; to possess lower levels of academic qualification; to stress the need for more time (especially for building rapport, explaining cultural factors, and explaining technical detail); to have experienced disrespect from practitioners; to value pre- and post-session discussion; and to desire more strongly to find alternative employment.

Analysis of qualitative data

Three major, though necessarily overlapping, themes emerged from examining the written responses to the open-ended section of the questionnaire.*

Theme one: skills to manage the job

Many participants wrote about the skills required by interpreters, which are varied and numerous; the knowledge and experience needed is extensive.

> Now I have knowledge of not just being an interpreter, but now I have knowledge of working with mentally disturbed people, vulnerable and desperate people, people from all over the world, learned about their culture, religion, political orders in their countries etc. I learned about legal and immigration law in this country and about all aspects in the community in general.
>
> (P58)

The linguistic skills required are also considerable. Interpreters need to be able to speak at least two languages fluently so that they can give a precise and accurate translation. Ideally, they should be able to convey the emotional affect implied through the choice of specific words in both languages.

> Translating for me is more of a hobby that I enjoy by finding out how to best express sentences from the one language to the other, without loss of any of the precise meaning.
>
> (P32)

The interpreter needs to be able to juggle the two conversants' speech, understanding the meaning and intent behind the communication, sometimes memorising long explanations, perhaps interrupting to ask the speaker to pause.

---

* Illustrative extract material in this section is reproduced verbatim, and referenced by Participant number.

Other comments indicated the need to be adaptable in order to cope with the many different circumstances under which interpreting is required. In order to describe the personal qualities and interpersonal skills demanded, adjectives were used such as *tactful, non-judgemental, intuitive, empathic, objective, supportive, diplomatic, reassuring, tolerant, intelligent,* and *patient.* Other prerequisites listed were common sense and the ability to inspire confidence.

> All interpreters should not only be excellent linguists but perceptive, sensitive and versatile people with plenty of experience and very good communication skills. Values and attitudes that are flexible and un-biased and open attitudes to race, culture, gender, politics and age or beliefs.
>
> (P26)

Such was the sort of person specification participants demanded of themselves! In order to facilitate rich discussion between the two speakers, the importance of building good rapport was also emphasised.

> The normal thing a good interpreter does is to introduce him or herself to the client in the client's dialect and if necessary his or her cultural way of greetings.
>
> (P7)

Interpreters may be required tactfully to interrupt a speaker if they notice the client or the practitioner looking confused, to help establish an atmosphere of trust, to explain cultural differences in behaviour, and to provide a middle ground for negotiation without offending the pride of either speaker. Also involved, is the ability to cope with clients who provide monosyllabic answers or rushed explanations, who attempt to manipulate them, or give constant contradictions.

> I found it hard to stop the client talking, as the sentences were all connected.
>
> (P38)

Some practitioners lack training and do not know how to adjust their technique in order to enable effective work to proceed.

Typical items include not being aware they must speak in short, clear sentences; not ensuring the interpreter can see their mouth when talking; and trying to hurry an interview, not recognising sessions will take considerably longer when conducted through an interpreter. The practitioner may also resent the interpreter's presence. Dealing with these aspects calls upon skills that are strictly speaking unnecessary, and which may go unrecognised.

> The practitioner often has no idea how complex and delicate the work is, and how skilled and tactful and expert an interpreter has to be. Practitioners (in all confidence) can sometimes resent the interpreter and the fact that he/she requires an interpreter is seen as a slight/threat to the practitioner's authority and status. This has to be approached with patience and tolerance by an 'aware' interpreter. On the other hand some practitioners are quick to appreciate and acknowledge the value of an interpreter and the role's usefulness.
>
> (P26)

Being well versed in the customs and practices of the two cultures also involves familiarity with their institutions, organisations and procedures; some understanding of the relevant historical, political, social and religious issues; and awareness of etiquette and taboos that are likely to influence the behaviour of the two speakers.

> Certain questions cannot be applied or approached without first considering the cultural differences.
>
> (P28)

Understanding too may be required of complex technical issues such as disease processes, medical investigations, form filling, and legal procedures.

> [I had to] make sure client understands implications of court verdict. Whatever may be the decision. In one case, client thought she is getting residency rights for her daughter. In fact she was denied these rights. Client was very upset.
>
> (P15)

Theme Two: Difficulties experienced, which hinder the exercise of those skills

Many responses indicated that participants often felt generally unappreciated. Frequently, for example, practitioners allow interpreters the sort of preparation time appropriate to working solely in English, ignoring their main role of accurately translating and communicating:

> At a particular court hearing a twenty page affidavit was shoved into my hand five minutes prior to going before the judge and, I was asked to explain same to client. I complained to the judge, who gave me a further half hour. Interpreters should be given any such material a few days before in order to get a chance to look up any technical terminology which we do not use in our ordinary daily conversations. People who spring wodges of material to be translated instantaneously are rude, disrespectful and cruel.
>
> (P20)

The tendency among practitioners of failing to inform interpreters of the intricacies of cases before the session begins can make it very difficult for them to establish rapport with the client. Some practitioners excuse this failing in the name of professional practice.

> Confidentiality is used as an excuse by many practitioners who only give interpreters the time, date and venue and not even the client's name. I feel only polite to be able to say: 'Good morning Mrs Ahmed' for instance. The total lack of preparation only leads to a longer interview.
>
> (P20)

> Practitioner and interpreter need to look at sensitive issues first and determine how they are best approached in order not to put the client in an embarrassing situation, especially if he is in front of a native speaker (fellow countryman).
>
> (P28)

Most participants attributed these failings to practitioners' attitudes towards themselves as interpreters, and their work.

The most difficult aspect of my work is no respect towards me, I am treated like I have no right to be at interview, that I am nobody, that I have no knowledge of what I do for my living, that I am part of the problem not part of the solution.

(P58)

They acknowledged that practitioners' attitudes varied from one situation to another. On one occasion they might be treated as a vital mediator and a crucial member of the team, while on another, they felt they were

. . . tolerated as a necessary evil.

(P59)

A further often unacknowledged aspect of the interpreting work was mentioned: it is emotionally demanding. Interpreters are rarely provided with any training or support systems to help deal with these demands.

. . . if it was really bad news you were interpreting it would be down to you how to pass this bad news and that makes me feel bad more than the practitioner as I am speaking directly to the client.

(P31)

In addition, another participant described how, when working with refugees, their situation brought back vivid memories of her own experiences, which she found difficult to cope with. The difficulty with remaining objective was compounded by factors such as:

[I] was their only link to the new society and system and they became very dependent.

(P53)

The addition of emotional involvement to the more obvious translation role of the interpreter's work was sensed partly to be yet another unnecessary intrusion and yet partly to be an unavoidable aspect. One participant felt it to be 'totally unnecessary' for an interpreter, but she did 'not know how to avoid' this sort of situation. Another felt that the distress consequent upon such involvement was unavoidable 'unless there was a strong support system'. The idea was mooted by another participant of forming self-help groups to provide the opportunity to debrief on some of the more distressing sessions.

Some participants wrote about working in a totally freelance capacity (as opposed to using the interpreting organisation as their 'agent'). Being completely freelance exacerbated problems of lack of continuity with clients – for instance, they might work once with a client at the beginning of a court case, then have no further contact at all.

> The client tends not to be completely open because there is a third person present, and in such circumstances, many things will be left out by the client. To avoid this situation, it would be preferable if the same interpreter is used often.
>
> (P4)

The practical organisation of interpreters' day-to-day employment provided a further source of stress – particularly, maintaining an 'on call' availability in the face of the unpredictability of work, of its variable time of day, and location. Metropolitan transport problems meant sometimes arriving late – or arriving on time only to find the client or the practitioner not yet arrived. Occasionally there would be no work for weeks on end, then the requirement to work long hours for days together. Not surprisingly, they reported being unable to rely on interpreting as a sole source of income. This sort of stress was responsible for losses to the pool of experienced workforce.

> It is not easy to make a living through working as an interpreter therefore most people leave the job completely.
>
> (P8)

When participants worked freelance (i.e. were employed direct by the services), payment was reported as habitually delayed, sometimes by months, as were travel expenses. And the level of remuneration was considered to be an inadequate reward for the skills and demands involved.

> The pay simply does not match the skill, intensity and challenge of the job . . . Much more recognition and awareness of the work we do is essential.
>
> (P26)

To the inadequacy of financial recognition, one or two participants added the lack of a career structure to the list of deficiencies experienced in their work – what was needed was a thorough assessment of applicants; initial and on-going training; being awarded a recognised professional status; and working within an established code of practice.

Theme three: role conflicts experienced in the job

Almost all participants recognised the primacy of language translation in their role as interpreters. The degree of primacy accorded to providing an impartial translation varied in what they wrote, from:

> The Interpreter is there for one reason only: to make communication possible and to enable the two parties to exchange the correct and precise information.
>
> (P61)

> Strictly speaking the role of the interpreter is to translate language . . . but it is often necessary, useful or desirable for the interpreter to have an extended role . . . e.g., to help, befriend, represent the client or communicate on their behalf.
>
> (P56)

Role conflict may thus arise for those interpreters who sense that good practice requires them to combine the impartial accuracy aspect of the work, with these further aspects involving, for example, befriending or advocacy. One participant recounted how she came across the need to extend her role: increasingly, she found she needed to:

> Understand the difficulties faced by the political refugees in the UK to present their cases. To understand their psychological traumas and their confusion, their fear, etc.
>
> (P42)

However, another wrote the following caution:

[It is important that you] do not overstep boundaries; you are a mouthpiece/facilitator, not a doctor.

(P33)

Many participants, therefore, reported their awareness of having to combine and balance aspects of their role. Its extension was expressed as having to anticipate and clarify confusions, explain relevant issues, elucidate technical or procedural factors, give an impression of the emotions conveyed in the client's spoken and body language, and act as the client's advocate.

A major help in coping with the role confusion was identified as team working with practitioners, preparing for the session, and alerting the practitioner to the possibility of unavoidable role conflict situations. One participant hinted that such team working would mean that the distinction employed by this research project, between 'practitioner' and 'interpreter', might dissolve, as the two became simply regarded as two practitioners.

. . . preparation is the key, as far as I'm concerned. Interpreters should not be working in isolation but as part, however temporarily, of the team of practitioners.

(P20)

Concluding discussion

The data provided by the 64 participants give a first-hand but not complete picture of the experience and role of interpreters. Several features of the research have to be acknowledged while considering the results. (i) The 21 per cent return rate is lower than the commonly expected 30–40 per cent. Were the 236 non-returners apathetic and demoralised? How would their responses have altered the picture obtained? (ii) Did the use of the interpreter organisation to frank and mail the questionnaires, plus its enclosed letter, have a biasing effect on the data gathered? Were the recipients willing to trust that their information would be wholly confidential? (iii) The questionnaire ignored both the interpreter organisation and the service agencies; nevertheless, as the employing organisations they cannot fail to be valid parts of the system involved.

These constraints admitted, the present results represent an initial empirical attempt to document what interpreters themselves have to say about their work. It is arguable that a single agency focus would have been advisable, but this research questioned interpreters about the whole span of experience of their work, rather than specifically about their contact with one service. Since all said they worked for multiple services, we believe that the wide focus we adopted has accessed more typical experience. The results and analysis of this experience very much speak for themselves (for a fuller discussion see Granger, 1996). However, the two major comments which follow attempt to develop what we found.

First, threaded through much of the data are several apparent contradictions, the most striking being that, while the interpreters reported a very high level of job satisfaction, many of them were keen to find another job. However, they gave many instances of dissatisfaction at these practices *not* being followed, making it difficult for them to carry out their role:

- frustration at not having professional status, and feeling excluded from the professional team
- extensive skills and expertise not recognised in terms of status and pay
- unlike practitioners, little support or supervision offered to cope with stressful aspects of the work.

The practicalities of the job were also difficult. They had no set routine or continuity; they were required to adapt to the greatly differing needs of various services situated all over London and the surrounding region; some were required to be available 24-hours a day while most get no more than 4 hours' employment a week. For some, this was compounded by being paid irregularly, and waiting for long periods to receive travel expenses.

It is not altogether surprising therefore that the majority was keen to find alternative employment. On the one hand, working as an interpreter could be seen as a reasonable short-term part-time job, to help finance further studies for example. The irregular and often antisocial hours would fit in conveniently and the individual would be able to make good use of their bilingual skills without being required to take any specific training. On the other hand, the working conditions are often so fraught that it is difficult not to conclude that some action needs to be taken.

Should this action be a simple adjustment to present conditions, or a thorough overhaul? The general thrust of the 'recommendations' drawn from the literature, and many of the comments from the present study, is towards a formal training, with associated higher levels of pay for qualified staff, and adherence to a Code of Practice.

Other considerations may however favour continuing with a haphazard system. It is our contention that the current data may represent an ambiguity sensed by the interpreters when considering this dilemma. For example, there is a recommendation in the literature concerning the importance of matching interpreters with clients in a culturally appropriate manner. This was not supported by the participants' quantitative data – yet their qualitative data show every indication of the high regard they give to cultural sensitivity. It is possible that interpreters in theory agree with such 'matching', but in practice feel that it contains the unspoken corollary that the very low number of hours' work they are offered each week might become even lower.

The variable, *length of service*, and the scores on the various other factors which were significantly associated with it, seemed at first sight to point to the possibility that those supporting the career structure 'path' were the more experienced interpreters. Those who had less experience seemed to be concentrating upon other goals (many of them were studying for further professional qualifications). These latter might be more inclined to aim at 'tweaking' the present system to rid it of its worst aggravations. However, it was the more experienced workers who gave the higher, more extreme ratings on the variable *desire alternative employment*.

It might be that those with more experience had more insight into the complexity of the role and were more aware of the need – for example – to have adequate time to prepare for a session and to establish good rapport with the client. These longer serving inter-preters would therefore feel more frustration when the recommen-dations for good practice were ignored. Worn down by such experiences together with the frustration of not having their skills recognised, they might well express a greater desire for alternative employment. There is a risk that those lost from the workforce pool would be from its most experienced sector.

Second, there seemed to us to be a distinction to be made between those employment difficulties that may be thought of as unneedful, and those that are inherent to the job – although the distinction would not be categorical. For instance, there may be an 'inherent' level of embarrassment when sexual issues have to be discussed through an interpreter, but it would presumably be possible not to add unnecessarily to this level – as in the case of one woman who described how she had had to interpret in such circumstances between a male practitioner and a male client.

Adoption of a Code of Practice would guard against such situations. Any Code would probably conflict with the preferences of individual practitioners, and be resisted by different institutions already operating under considerable financial and time pressures. It would however be a practical step towards avoiding unnecessary hindrances to good practice.

A well-structured training and support system would be an important item within such a Code. Another would be a job description – though the diversity of roles and required skills from one setting to another give even this seemingly simple task unavoidable complexity. There is also the cost to purchasers of interpreter services, which cannot be ignored. Perhaps the challenge of the present study's data is less to pinpoint the dilemma interpreters may find themselves in ('Do you want a career structure, or don't you?') and more to start asking ourselves as part of the system, which includes the interpreters, questions about dilemmas affecting the whole team because of their economic implications. Perhaps the failure of the present study to include the wider employing organisations either side of *the interpreter*, *the client* and *the practitioner*, was more serious than we realised.

The quality of service offered to individuals from different cultural and linguistic backgrounds is unlikely to match that provided for English-speaking clients if the role of interpreters is not allowed to evolve and develop. But this will not happen without adequate financial backing.

Acknowledgements

The authors warmly acknowledge the facilitation and advice of Hitesh Raval and Rachel Tribe in the research described, the interpreter's organisation involved, and the freely given help of the interpreters who participated.

References

Boyle, M., Baker, M., Bennett, E. and Charman, T. (1993) 'Selection for clinical psychology courses: a comparison of applicants from ethnic minority and majority groups to University of East London'. *Clinical Psychology Forum*, 56: 9–13.

Cox, J. (1977) 'Aspects of transcultural psychiatry'. *British Journal of Psychiatry*, 130: 211–221.

Faust, M. and Drickey, M. (1986) 'Working with interpreters'. *Journal of Family Practice*, 22: 131–138.

Freed, A. (1988) 'Interviewing through an interpreter'. *Social Work*, 33: 315–319.

Good, B. and Good, D. (1981) 'The meaning of symptoms: a cross-cultural hermeneutic model for clinical practice'. In L. Eisenberg and A. Kleinman (eds), *The Relevance of Social Science for Medicine*. Dordrecht, Holland: Reidel Publishing.

Granger, E. (1996) 'An investigation into the role and work experience of the interpreter'. Unpublished doctoral thesis, University of East London.

Harvey, M. (1984) 'Family therapy with deaf persons: the systematic utilization of an interpreter'. *Family Process*, 23: 205–213.

Hillier, S., Loshak, R., Marks, F. and Rahman, S. (1994) 'An evaluation of child psychiatric services for Bangladeshi parents'. *Journal of Mental Health*, 3: 327–337.

Kaufert, J. and Koolage, W. (1984) 'Role conflict among "cultural brokers": the experience of native Canadian medical interpreters'. *Social Science Medicine*, 18: 283–286.

Kline, F., Adrian, A. and Spevak, M. (1980) 'Clients evaluate therapists'. *Archives of General Psychiatry*, 31: 113–116.

Owan, T. (1985) *South East Asian Mental Health: Treatment, Prevention, Services, Training and Research*. Rockville, MD: National Institute for Mental Health.

Raval, H. (1996) 'A systemic perspective on working with interpreters'. *Clinical Child Psychology and Psychiatry*, 1: 29–43.

Roe, D. and Roe, C. (1991) 'The third party: using interpreters for the deaf in counselling situations'. *Journal of Mental Health Counselling*, 13: 91–105.

Roy, C.B. (1992) 'A socio-linguistic analysis of the interpreter's role in simultaneous talk in a face-to-face interpreted dialogue'. *Sign Language Studies*, 5: 21–61.

Saunders, M. and Broune, J. (1992) 'Working with interpreters'. London Interpreting Project (LIP) workshop handouts.

Shackman, J. (1984) *The Right to be Understood: A Handbook on Working with, Employing, and Training Community Interpreters*. Cambridge: National Extension College.

Stansfield, M. (1981) 'Psychological issues in mental health interpreting RID'. *Interpreting Journal*, 1: 18–31.

Tribe, R. (1991) 'Bi-cultural workers – bridging the gap or damming the flow?' Paper to 11th International Conference of Centres, Institutions and Individuals concerned with the care of victims of organised violence: Health, political repression and human rights. Santiago, Chile.

Chapter 8

Applying theoretical frameworks to the work with interpreters

Hitesh Raval

Introduction

Interpreters in their role as cultural brokers and culture consultants can help clinicians to develop a more sophisticated understanding of the service user's mental health difficulties within a culturally appropriate framework. Interpreters also help give meaning to the communication between the clinician and the service user, in ways that the two of them can access. In order to develop a therapeutic relationship, the clinician and the service user need to negotiate issues relating to the cultural differences between them (Cheatham et al, 1993). The multi-cultural issues, which need negotiating, include those related to differences associated with age, gender, language, ethnicity, religion, socio-economic situation, trauma, cultural identity, and sexual orientation. With the interpreter this becomes a three-way negotiation.

Ecological frameworks

Geertz (1973) has defined culture as a web of meanings. Falicov (1995) defines culture as those sets of shared worldviews, meanings and adaptive behaviours derived from simultaneous membership and participation in a multiplicity of contexts (e.g. urban, rural, suburban setting; language, age, gender, cohort, family configuration, race, ethnicity, religion, nationality, socio-economic status, employment, education, occupation, sexual orientation, political ideology, migration, and acculturation). The groups produced by the different combinations of 'simultaneous memberships' and 'participation in multiple contexts', are thought to be more varied, fluid, unpredictable and shifting than groups defined by using an ethnic-focused approach. Falicov takes four broad comparative parameters in order to develop a cultural understanding of families through basically an ecological model:

1. Ecological context (including community, work, school).
2. Migration/acculturation context (which is associated with the uprooting of meaning). This uprooting of meaning may be internal (resulting from separation and reunions, traumas and crises, grief, mourning, disorientating anxieties, cultural identity), or external (language, social networks, institutions, values).
3. Family-life cycle (norms/ideals) as seen through stages (content, age appropriate timing, sequence) and transitions (change mechanisms, timing, rituals and rites).
4. Family organisation as seen through dominant dyads (husband–wife within a nuclear family or child–parent within an extended family) and boundaries.

Smail (1990) has proposed a theoretical model, which also places a greater emphasis on environmental influences and power as a way of contextualising human distress. He views power (i.e. coercive, economic, and ideological) as having the potential to exert a benign or malign influence on an individual. His version of a post-behavioural clinical psychology framework gives consideration to distal influences (e.g. culture, class, ideology) and proximal influences (e.g. family relations, personal relationships, work situation, domestic situation, education), and how these can impact on people's lives through mediating processes such as feelings, beliefs, metaphors, and symptoms. Smail envisages professional help being provided to service users at the personal level (e.g. clarification of the problem, comfort and encouragement for the individual), the social level (e.g. welfare, education, self-help, community support), or the political level (e.g. changing the way clinical psychology services are provided). Speigal (1982) has proposed a similar ecological model, which contextualises human distress within the interconnections between the psychological and somatic experiences or expressions of distress, in connection with other people, the cultural and societal context, and the environment. Such models help develop interventions at both the individual and contextual level. For example, the expression of distress following a physical assault may be manifested at the somatic (e.g. panic attacks) or psychological level (e.g. depressed mood), and perhaps at a community level (e.g. general unease and worry about such attacks within the neighbourhood). A successful intervention may need to address a number of factors such as helping the individual client (e.g. relaxation training or medication), securing retribution (e.g. successful police intervention to secure custodial sentence), or helping the individual get re-housed.

Ecological models have their strength in being able to take account of the contextual factors in understanding human distress, and they provide an affinity with culturally traditional models of human illness and well being. They provide a good fit for many communities with traditional understandings about illness based on environmental and spiritual beliefs. However, ecological models are theoretically weak in not being able to define or test empirically the causal pathways and relationships between the contextual factors and an individual's psychological distress. Interpreters bring their cultural perspective to the work and can play an important role as cultural brokers. Developing ways to access the connections between context, language, metaphors, and meaning provides clinicians with culturally appropriate ways to help service users (Krause, 1995; Maitra and Miller, 1996; Woodcock, 1995).

Multi-cultural frameworks

More recently some authors have taken the position that all theories are culturally embedded and therefore can only be understood in relation to the context in which they were produced (Cheatham et al, 1993; Sue et al, 1996). Falicov (1995) argues that theories, which take up universalist (i.e. generic theory or understanding can explain most things about a family), particularist (i.e. each family can only be understood in their unique way), or ethnic-focused positions (i.e. a family can best be understood on the basis of their ethnicity), are limited in the understanding that they can generate about families. For Falicov, a multi-dimensional position needs to be taken in order to address the complexities not covered by the other three positions.

In developing their theory of multi-cultural counselling and therapy (MCT), Sue et al (1996) have put forward the following propositions:

1. MCT is a meta-theory of counselling and psychotherapy (i.e. it has a framework which allows different theoretical models to be applied and integrated whenever possible).
2. Both the clinician's and the service user's identities are formed and embedded in multiple levels of life experiences (individual, group, universal) and context (individual, family, cultural). Psychological interventions should take greater account of the service user's experiences in relation to his or her context.
3. The cultural identity development of the clinician and the service user, in the context of the power differentials associated with this, plays an important role in establishing a therapeutic relationship.
4. The effectiveness of MCT is enhanced when the clinician defines intervention goals and uses modes of treatment that are consistent with the life experiences and cultural values of the service user.
5. MCT theory stresses the importance of multiple helping roles, which have been developed across different cultural groups and societies, besides the idea of one-to-one counselling. At times the helping role may involve interventions aimed at the larger social units or systems.
6. MCT theory helps the service user develop a greater awareness about him or herself in relation to the context. This results in therapy that takes context into consideration when planning interventions, and therapy that draws on traditional methods of healing which are used across all cultures.

The work of Cheatham et al (1993) and Sue et al (1996) is helpful in providing a guiding framework for thinking about the stance that one might take when doing cross-cultural counselling. However, as a theoretical framework it lacks sufficient clarity about how it would generate testable causal explanations about psychological problems. It gives no explanations about how the duration and course of the problems is influenced by the contextual factors and the multi-cultural issues. Also, MCT does not contain an adequate amount of detail to determine how theoretically opposed models can be integrated into the one framework.

Theoretical models dealing with meaning

Cronen et al (1982) have put forward a framework that also takes account of context in relation to meanings that are created by people. They have proposed a hierarchy of contexts starting with culture, society, family, individual, behaviour, and speech acts. They argue that the same observation (or action) may be given a different meaning depending on which context is being used in order to give meaning to that observation. Within their framework they state that a change of meaning at a higher-level context can lead to it changing through the lower-level contexts. Changes in meaning at a lower contextual level may not always readily lead to changes in meaning at a higher contextual level. For example, a child seen as a troublemaker in the classroom may find it hard to be seen differently by his teacher by changing his behaviour, but may be viewed very differently after a doctor has diagnosed an illness in the child.

From a constructivist position the meanings and understanding generated from observation and interaction with the environment are thought to be unique to any individual (Andersen, 1987; Efran et al, 1988; Hoffman, 1988; Tomm, 1988). This position argues that individual understandings and constructions of the world are unique to any individual, and that people make sense of their environment by developing a functional fit or understanding. Individual realities are thought to be constituted in language, and knowledge is thought to be constructed and hence relative (Anderson and Goolishian, 1988). Individual action is thought to be less predictable, and meaning construction is thought to be context dependent. In contrast, social constructionism takes the position that meanings are socially created through discourse (Burr, 1995; McNamee and Gergen, 1992). Certain discourses are thought to become dominant in relation to others, having a powerful effect on how people are able to experience and give meaning to their actions and the actions of others. Again this position highlights the relative nature of meaning and the importance of language in the creation of reality.

Kaufert (1990) has developed a psycho-biomedical model for medical interpreting, which draws out the importance of paying attention to the individual contextual factors and beliefs about illness held by the interpreter, clinician, and service user. He suggests that initially each one of them may hold very different

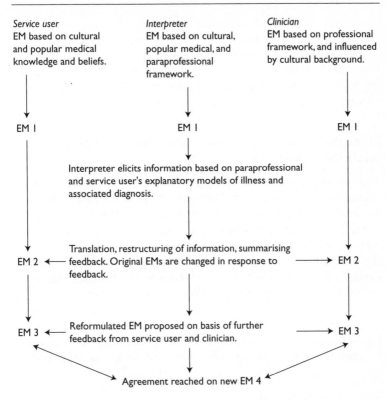

Figure 8.1   Dynamics of interactions between Explanatory Models (EMs) of clinicians, interpreters and service users

explanatory models about the service user's illness based on traditional or lay theories of illness (with the clinician also drawing on medical knowledge). A process of negotiation occurs through the interpreter, which enables the clinician and the service user to come to a mutually agreeable and consensual explanatory model (EM) of the service user's illness. The interpreter is working largely as a cultural broker during this process, but would be influenced by his or her own explanatory model. The process associated with reaching the consensual explanatory model is given in Figure 8.1, which presents an adapted version of the Figure used by Kaufert (1990, p. 216). Difficulties are likely to arise when one or more of the three parties involved adhere to polarised or incompatible explanatory models about the service user's illness. The interpreter has to carry out sensitive cultural brokerage in helping the clinician and the service user reach a consensual explanatory model. The interpreter has to amplify, simplify, and change the semantic structure in order to facilitate shared understanding between the clinician and the service user, and will inevitably influence this process by his or her explanatory model.

Usefulness of the frameworks to the work with interpreters

The cross-cultural and ecological frameworks are helpful in providing clinicians with a number of ways in which to develop a better understanding of the impact of the service user's context on the difficulties being experienced by the service user. There is also an emphasis on the clinician having to give greater consideration to the service user's perspective in order not to impose the clinician's explanatory model on to the user. Hopefully, this encourages the clinician to develop more culturally appropriate explanatory models of illness and ways of helping the service user. Interpreters play an important role as translators, cultural brokers, and cultural intermediaries. The ecological and multi-cultural frameworks make it easier to incorporate interpreters more broadly into the work.

The significance of context

Context plays a significant part in how people experience psychological difficulties, and how these are understood by the clinician. Cultural beliefs, class, gender, etc. all form a basis from which personal and shared narratives are formed about what are culturally acceptable ways of experiencing distress; ways that are allowed within a particular family or community group for being able to exhibit such distress (and those that are unacceptable), and the types of help that are sanctioned or made possible to access. An interpreter can play an important role in helping the clinician determine some of the above subtleties when working with an individual or family in need of his or her help. An understanding of such factors can help the clinician develop an informed and culturally appropriate intervention. For example, the successful implementation of a behavioural intervention with a child may be contingent on addressing the parents' spiritual causal explanations about the child's difficult behaviour at school. The parents may hold a strong belief that their child is possessed by an evil spirit, and that the problem will only be 'cured' by carrying out a religious ritual to exorcise the evil spirit. Until these issues have been satisfactorily addressed and taken on board, the parents are unlikely to engage in an intervention plan where the emphasis is on getting them to change their management strategies with the child. The interpreter can therefore play an important role in informing the clinician about factors that may need to be considered in developing a culturally appropriate understanding of the problem, and a successful intervention that is embedded within and consistent with the family's beliefs.

The interpreter will be bringing his or her own context into the work. This too has to be understood and incorporated into the work, as much as the context that the clinician will be bringing into the work and therapeutic relationship with the service user. The need for the clinician and interpreter to become familiar and understanding of each other's context is thus of paramount importance. For effective co-working both the interpreter and the clinician need to feel comfortable with where each of them is coming from. Difficulties and tensions often arise in this work when such understanding has not been developed. It is hard for the interpreter to represent the clinician and be a cultural broker for the clinician, if for example the interpreter does not have a context or rationale for why a particular line of questioning is being adopted. If the interpreter has very little experience of mental health work, many of the concepts underlying the questions that are used in an interview will make little sense. The interpreter would find it hard, if not impossible, to translate questions that do not make sense or that cannot be translated verbatim, but which require an explanation before the service user is in a position to answer them in a meaningful way that generates information which the clinician can use. Certain questions may seem to come out of the blue given that the interpreter will not have had access to the clinician's line of thinking, which led to asking that particular question at a given point in time. Other questions may be personally difficult for the interpreter to ask the service user, such as intimate questions about sexual behaviour or abuse. These types of difficulties can be made easier by allocating discussion time prior to starting a piece of work.

The personhood of the interpreter is an important factor that will play an important part in how well it is possible to engage with a service user. There has to be time built into the work for providing the interpreter with an opportunity to explore this in the work with the clinician, and be given space to process the emotional impact of the work. As people, interpreters will be equally moved by and resonate with the personal life stories that are brought to the work by the service user. They are not immune to this by being positioned as a neutral translator by the clinician. Co-working and support play an important part in this type of work.

The significance of multi-cultural theories

Another tension that arises in this work is when the clinician's theories no longer seem to fit with the information or causal explanation being provided by the service user. In frustration it is easy to become dismissive of the service user or the interpreter when faced with information that does not seem to be making sense. The multi-dimensional position offered by Falicov (1995) offers the clinician the opportunity to remain open minded to alternative possible explanations and beliefs about the problem. The help offered by the clinician will only be useful if a level of consensus can be reached between the clinician, service user, and the interpreter.

The interpreter plays a useful role in helping the clinician develop knowledge and understanding of the service user's difficulties. At both a broader and individual level, the interpreter is ideally placed to provide the service user and the clinician with a contextual framework that facilitates the bringing forth of an understanding of the difficulties of the service user and possible explanations for it. This type of cultural brokerage is an important part of the process of reaching a consensus about the problem, and in reacting upon culturally agreed goals as a means of alleviating this. It also helps the clinician from holding too rigidly to a 'universalist' position about human distress. The interpreter can help prevent the clinician and the service user from drawing back into their strongly held beliefs, and thereby reaching an impasse.

A multi-cultural position encourages the clinician to explore how one's own cultural identity development, and that of others, can have a significant bearing on the successful engagement with a service user and a positive therapeutic outcome. For example, working with a young female interpreter who has a stronger liberal cultural identity may make it difficult to create an engagement with a more traditional father in a family. An older authoritarian male clinician may also need to think through cultural identity issues if the young female interpreter is going to be able to develop an equitable co-working alliance with the clinician. Issues of power may come to the fore particularly if aspects of the disempowerment, which are being experienced by the interpreter or the service user within their community context, are re-enacted in the process of the therapeutic encounter. An interpreter may feel too overwhelmed by a particular clinician in order to carry out the work effectively, or may become more explicitly challenging of the clinician in front of the service user in ways that are contrary to meeting the needs of the service user. Often clinicians do not allow for the 'thinking time' needed in order to negotiate and process issues, such as those described above with the interpreter, at the time of doing the work.

The significance of meanings

Working with language and meaning is a large component of therapeutic work in mental health. The contextual, constructivist and social constructionist frameworks help clinicians to place the interpreter as an important partner in the co-creation of a web of meanings. They also highlight how much is taken for granted in monolingual communication, and the important role that the interpreter has in rendering meaning and facilitating meaningful communication between the clinician and the service user. Although the ideal process proposed by Kaufert (1990) whereby an agreed consensus is reached is often difficult to attain in this kind of work, it is nonetheless one that clinicians should be aiming for.

In the three-way process of communication numerous meanings may well be attributed to what at first seems like a straightforward piece of information sharing or transfer, particularly as the communication is having to take place across several levels of cultural and language systems. Conversations can only be made sense of in the broader context, and the more specific context of the particular relationship within which the two people talking are choosing to define themselves. Much of the initial phase of working with an interpreter involves negotiating the definitions or parameters that each person is willing to participate in within the context of the therapeutic relationship. Unless this phase is negotiated successfully all the other phases of the work cannot take place smoothly. Again, the amount of time that is needed in this early phase of the work in order to clarify such issues cannot be under-estimated. Chances of misunderstandings are likely to increase if this basic groundwork has not been done.

Acknowledging that meanings and realities are created through conversations thus leads the clinician away from holding onto 'universalist' positions. The meanings and insights into the problem that will have relevance for the service user will be those that are derived from the context of the service user, that make sense and hold a certain level of validity within his or her understanding of the world. This does not mean that the interpreter's or clinician's knowledge and ideas will have little use, but in order to be useful they have to make sense within the service user's life experiences and understandings of the world. The task for the interpreter becomes one of facilitating the therapeutic process such that this becomes possible. Again, for this kind of work to be done effec-tively, interpreters need to go beyond the literal translation. The extent to which they can do this successfully comes back to the role they play in the work, and needs to take into account how the interpreter's own context will influence the meaning or under-standing that is co-created. For example, if an interpreter sees a mental health interview as being tasked with the granting or denial of asylum status within the context of a home office interview, the questions requiring translation may assume a very different status, than if the same questions were being asked as part of a routine outpatient appointment. The context in which the interview is taking place may have a significant bearing on the process of the interview, and the personal impact that this may have on the interpreter carrying out this piece of work.

Concluding remarks

Whilst the frameworks described in this chapter begin to provide a helpful starting point, further work is needed in order to create a firmer theoretical foundation from which to develop clinical practice utilising interpreters. The chapters that now follow have drawn on the theoretical frameworks described in this chapter, to a greater or lesser degree, in looking at ways of developing good clinical practice utilising interpreters. Each of the authors has described practice issues that are grounded in rich experience of working with interpreters across a variety of different types of service user groups.

References

Anderson, H. and Goolishian, H. (1988) 'Human systems as linguistic systems: preliminary and evolving ideas about the implications for clinical theory'. *Family Process*, 27: 371–393.

Andersen, T. (1987) 'The reflecting team: dialogue and meta-dialogue in clinical work'. *Family Process*, 26: 415–428.

Burr, V. (1995) *An Introduction to Social Constructionism*. London: Routledge.

Cheatham, H., Ivey, A., Ivey, M. and Simek-Morgan, L. (1993) 'Multicultural counselling and therapy. Changing the foundations of the field'. In A. Ivey, M. Ivey and L. Simek-Morgan (eds), *Counselling and Psychotherapy: A Multicultural Perspective*. London: Allyn and Bacon Publishers, Chapter 5.

Cronen, V., Johnson, K. and Lannahan, J. (1982) 'Paradoxes double binds and negative loops: an alternative theoretical perspective'. *Family Process*, 21: 91–112.

Efran, J.S., Lukens, R.J. and Lukens, M.D. (1988) 'Constructivism: what's in it for you?' *Networker*, Sep–Oct: 27–35.

Falicov, C.J. (1995) 'Training to think culturally: a multidimensional comparative framework'. *Family Process*, 34: 373–388.

Geertz, C. (1973) *The Interpretation of Culture*. London: Fontana Publishers.

Hoffman, L. (1988) 'Constructing realities: an art of lenses'. *Family Process*, 29: 1–12.

Kaufert, J.M. (1990) 'Sociological and anthropological perspectives on the impact of interpreters on clinician/client communication'. *Sante Culture Health*, VII(2–3): 209–235.

Krause, I.-B. (1995) 'Personhood, culture and family therapy'. *Journal of Family Therapy*, 17: 363–382.

McNamee, S. and Gergen, K.J. (1992) *Therapy as Social Construction*. London: Sage Publications.

Maitra, B. and Miller, A. (1996) 'Children, families and therapists: clinical considerations and ethnic minority cultures'. In K.N. Dwivedi and V.P. Varma (eds), *Meeting the Needs of Ethnic Minority Children*. London: Jessica Kingsley Publishers, pp. 111–129.

Smail, D. (1990) 'Design for a post-behaviourist clinical psychology'. *Clinical Psychology Forum*, 22: 2–10.

Speigal, J. (1982) 'An ecological model of ethnic families'. In M.

McGoldrick, J. Pearce and J. Giordano (eds), *Ethnicity and Family Therapy*. London: Guilford Press.

Sue, D.W., Ivey, A.E. and Pedersen, P.B. (1996) 'A theory of multicultural counselling and therapy'. Pacific Grove, CA: Brooks/Cole Publishing Company.

Tomm, K. (1988) 'Interventive interviewing: Part III. Intending to ask lineal, circular, strategic, or reflexive questions?'. *Family Process*, 27: 1–15.

Woodcock, J. (1995) 'Healing rituals with families in exile'. *Journal of Family Therapy*, 17: 397–404.

Chapter 9

From postmen to makers of meaning: a model for collaborative work between clinicians and interpreters

Philip Messent

Amato was an Italian author who migrated to New Zealand, where he wrote his fiction in English. He describes in his short story, *One of the Titans* (1992, p. 117), an encounter in Italy between an Italian and an English speaking bank-teller. The Italian, considering migrating to Australia, had asked the bank-teller what Australia was like. 'Si', she had said, 'La moneta é buona,' which, to an Italian, meant only 'Yes, the coin is good-hearted.' The bank-teller's meaning only became clear to the Italian some time later. As Amato goes on to comment: 'no Italian could understand unless he first understood what "Yes, the money is good" could mean.'

Interpreting goes beyond translating spoken sentences from one language to another, word for word. It demands a knowledge of the way in which both languages are used, which includes their idioms, their figures of speech, their metaphors, their similes, as well as the values, goals and communication styles of those individuals and groups using them. The irony in Amato's story is that his Italian migrant goes on to find the emphasis on the acquisition of money in his adopted homeland deeply alienating.

The myth of the interpreter as postman

Pearce (1989) suggests that the prevalent, though usually unarticulated, theory of communication in the west is that described by Miller (1986) as a 'post office' model of communication. The idea here is that even in a simple exchange between two people what is happening is that an idea occurs in one person's mind, it is 'wrapped' in words and sent off to the other person, who unwraps the words to discover the idea within. According to such a model the role of the interpreter would be simply to carry the idea from one person to the other, re-wrapping it en route in order that it should be understood clearly. Such a model would have it that words can straightforwardly 'stand for' the ideas they refer to, that we all share a common set of such ideas, and that the personhood of the interpreter has no impact upon the message being communicated. We do not after all see the personality of our postman as affecting in any way the meaning of the letters he delivers. Clinicians wishing for their communications to be translated word for word, who mistrust interpreters when their utterances do not seem to correspond in length or tone to their own, are in effect adopting such a model of communication.

Such a model however does not do justice to the complexity of what is going on in communication in several important respects. Wittgenstein (1953) demonstrated that there is no simple correspondence between words and the ideas that they express. We cannot meaningfully talk about a world of ideas that exist in a 'pure' form, that we all somehow have access to, using words merely as a secondary means of expression of such ideas. 'Meaning is use': we give our ideas meaning only by the words that we use, and by agreeing together about the meaning that we are going to give those words. When a European clinician meets a client recently arrived from rural Bangladesh, for example, the two of them will share neither a common language, nor this agreement about a common meaning system. Both might agree, for example, that the nature of their relationship is one of help, but they may have very different ideas about what such 'help' is likely to consist of.

An English-speaking child psychiatrist was interviewing a Bangladeshi family through an interpreter about their concerns about one of the children in the family. One of the parents asked her: 'What will happen if he doesn't get any better?' The psychiatrist replied: 'We will work together until we find a way of helping him get better.' The interpreter, rather than translating this statement, indicated to the psychiatrist that he did not think this statement would have much meaning to family members, and asked the psychiatrist's permission to explain to them what this 'working together' might involve. The interpreter knew that the parents' initial expectation of their consultation with the psychiatrist would be that she would make a diagnosis and then a medical intervention. They would not have any expectation of the need for themselves to be a part of the treatment process, involved in activities such as record-keeping and trying different ways of responding to their child, and the interpreter felt that he needed to spell out to them such expectations of the psychiatrist at this point in order to make her words intelligible. Thus translating one sentence involved a lengthy explanation, the interpreter making use of several years' experience of working in the agency to give a distillation of the sort of things that might be involved in this 'working together'.

The interpreter here needed to have a good working knowledge of the two languages, including their figures of speech, metaphors, similes and idioms, and he needed to appreciate that these did not simply translate from one language to the other. He needed to be familiar with the meaning systems of both clinician and family members – how they would hear each other's communications given their previous experience and beliefs, the kinds of techniques and approaches the psychiatrist might use, and the way in which these would be received. The interpreter had to interpret what he believed the clinician intended to communicate (based on the shared meaning system evolved over several years of working in the same agency) in a manner which he believed family members would be able to understand, make sense of, and welcome (based on their shared cultural meaning system).

Although this lack of a shared meaning system is particularly dramatic and stark in this circumstance, where the cultural difference between clinician and client is obvious, and the task of the interpreter particularly onerous), the very same difficulties occur where a culture is shared. It is equally true of white British families who come to a Child and Adolescent Mental Health Service for help that client and clinician will not begin with the same idea about what that help will consist of, and that if the contact is going to be productive, some shared meaning will have to be developed. And if the clinician is going to effectively 'join' (Minuchin and Fishman, 1981) with such a family, he/she will need to frame the nature of the help that is on offer in a manner that is sufficiently close to family members' ideas to be acceptable to them, in effect acting as his own interpreter. In all communication, but especially in therapeutic conversations, we are behaving as Pearce (1989) suggests more like poets than scientists. Rather than searching for words that 'truly' match an experience or an idea, we are looking more often for words, images, or metaphors that will reflect some aspect of an experience in a way that will be both true to the client's experience, and move the client on, by helping him/her to view the experience in a new way. Where a parent comes with complaints about a child's behaviour, seeing something as 'wrong' with their child, the clinician will be looking for ways of making sense of such behaviour differently: in a manner that is true to the parent's experience, but also allowing for the possibility of change.

Another important way in which the interpreter's role inevitably goes far beyond that of a postman is the way in which their personhood enters the relationship between the client and the professional agency. Interpreters will still be seen by clients as members of their community, more or less similar to them in terms of their origins, age and gender, and their communications understood in the light of these judgments. A very common question asked by Bangladeshi families is about the village or town that our interpreters and their families originate from. This seems to be a way of placing them, perhaps because such clients are looking for a personal connection, perhaps because they are wary about the confidentiality of their consultation. It was noticeable that a young Bangladeshi male interpreter, who had never been to Bangladesh and who represented himself as having little interest and few connections there, remained relatively distant and disconnected from family members during the therapeutic process (and thus was able to operate more like that mythical being, the 'pure' interpreter). The fact that it is the community in Bangladesh that is the first point of reference, indicates something about the importance for this community of the connections with families 'back home'. Later on in therapy families may also want to know about where interpreters live in the UK. This is likely to be relatively close to family members, in as much as the community here is clustered in certain areas of London. This may sound obvious but interpreters are often members of the same community as their clients, whereas therapists are mostly outsiders, living elsewhere and leading different lives from the clients they are providing a service for. Such interpreters can speak with real authority about managing the business of living as part of this community: dealing with racism, missing family members in Bangladesh, the mysteries of the education system, the housing system, and the major preoccupations of everyday life. If interpreters are instructed by clinicians, anxious about their own role, to limit their role strictly to translating what is being said, then a vast repertoire of knowledge and experience can be lost to the therapeutic process. Surely we should instead attempt to include such perspectives, which may connect power-fully with clients' worldviews in a way that is not possible for therapists from different cultures and communities.

A young Bangladeshi man married the eldest daughter in a family I had been working with for some time. He asked for advice about finding a job, and I referred him to our Bangladeshi interpreter, a man of mature years with much experience of managing the employment market in the UK, happy in the knowledge that the advice he got would be more relevant and acceptable than anything I could offer. This advice giving would at the same time further my therapeutic connectedness in my on-going work with the family in as much as the interpreter's advice was seen and valued by the wider family as a part of the service we were providing as a clinical team.

Making the most of it

Rennie (1998) even argues that in psychiatric treatment working with interpreters is so very difficult that 'effective therapy in such cases may be impossible to achieve'. The contrasting view articulated here is that interpreters will rarely prevent important information from being exchanged, and should rather be regarded as a potential asset, enriching the contact between client and clinician, as exemplified above, by their presence. One study, which demonstrates that interpreters need not have a negative effect upon the quality of at least a psychiatric diagnostic interview, was carried out by Farooq et al (1997), who compared the accuracy in terms of the diagnostic information gathered during adult psychiatric interviews via an interpreter with that gathered by a psychiatrist who spoke the relevant Asian language (Mirpuri). Although some minor qualitative differences were noted, there were no significant differences in terms of the facts regarded for these purposes as crucial (symptoms, family history, etc.). In fact there were more differences in the information gathered by the two psychiatrists jointly interviewing the English patients who were the control group, suggesting that individual differences between clinicians made more impact than the necessity or otherwise of using an interpreter.

One example of making positive therapeutic use out of the presence of an interpreter is discussed by Harvey (1984) in working with deaf persons, where the very presence of an interpreter can represent a challenge to the way in which one family is organising itself around the disability, ignoring the impact of the deafness. Simply by being a part of the therapeutic team, the interpreter is communicating to the client family that the therapeutic agency is viewing things in a way that is new for the family, treating the deafness as a disability which the agency is going to have to make special efforts to work with, to ensure the deaf person's full co-operation. The inclusion of an interpreter in this way contradicts the family's normal way of behaving towards the deaf person, thus challenging them to make more adaptations in their manner of communication with their deaf family member.

In a similar way having an interpreter present with an immigrant family in Britain is already communicating something about an agency's intentions and beliefs. Often in Bangladeshi families in Tower Hamlets, because of the pattern of migration and restrictions on women's role in communicating with external bodies, men and children are more fluent in English than women. Having an interpreter present allows for the possibility of women's views being heard and accorded respect in a way which in itself may be different from a family's normal organisation, encouraging other family members to view them in a new way, and allowing for the possibility of new solutions, in which women's power and authority is more acknowledged.

Interpreters will nearly always have specialist knowledge of the culture and religion they share with client families, knowledge which can be invaluable in therapeutic work. Very often inter-preters have provided me with extremely important insights about cultural rules and advice about the appropriateness of particular metaphors and tasks; for example, who might most appropriately be asked to talk to a 10-year-old boy about how to control his temper, or to a 15-year-old boy about managing his sexual urges. This is not to say, however, that such workers should be attributed the status of experts on their culture, tempting as it might be to do so. Many is the time that I have caught myself turning to an interpreter during a break when we have left the client family to consider what to do, to ask about cultural norms 'How do most Bangladeshi families deal with rebellious adolescents?', as if such norms were unchanging, easily accessible and universally acknowl-edged. In fact of course individual interpreters will have very different perspectives: as Farooq et al (1997) point out, interpreters may have very different cultural values to a client family. Rather than treating interpreters as all-knowing experts in their own culture, it seems to me more realistic to make use of their perspective in therapy as one amongst many that may be helpful to the family.

Rather than going away from families to ask such questions of interpreters in a separate conversation, it can be more productive to hold such discussions openly with the families involved, so that they have a range of different perspectives to draw from in thinking about problems and their solution.

A Bangladeshi father brought his 11-year-old eldest son for help. He had learning difficulties, and when at home would withdraw to his room, then go into an odd trance like state, in which he would speak to himself unintelligibly, and wet and soil himself. The father seemed resigned to this state of affairs, and my efforts to encourage him to stop his son withdrawing by engaging him more in family life at home had no effect. He would return for session after session, reporting the same pattern of behaviour in the same miserable yet resigned manner. His way of talking, however, changed dramatically when I began a discussion with him and our male interpreter about how he could teach his son to become a good Muslim, a task that was becoming increasingly urgent as the boy grew older. The father told us with real energy and spirit about his repeated and unavailing efforts to teach his son the first sentences from the Koran. Suddenly I was presented with a whole other side to this man, who I had previously seen as wholly uninvolved with his son. I invited the two Bangladeshi men, the interpreter and the client's father, to enlighten me about Muslim teaching on how people with learning difficulties could be expected to express their faith, and in the ensuing discussion a diversity of ideas emerged. This diversity seemed to help the father change his position so that he didn't view this recitation as the only way his son could express his faith, and his methods of engaging his son at home became more realistic and appropriate to his intellectual abilities. What was important in this discussion was that the interpreter offered some difference without ever implying that the father was wrong; indeed he was highly deferential about the father's religious expertise. It is in a climate of mutual respect of one another's knowledge and experience that different views and perspectives can be entertained.

With trained and experienced interpreters it becomes more possible to draw on their ideas and suggestions. The ability to reflect on how one's own context has a bearing on the work is another important skill for interpreters to be able to develop, as this prevents them from becoming too rigid in what they feel is going to be helpful to a family. Interpreters bring their personhood into the work and need to feel comfortable enough with the clinician's views and ideas in order to be able to convey these to the family.

I would see working with an interpreter as no more than a special example of the sort of co-working that is common in multidisciplinary teams, where two team members, often from different disciplines, collaborate in seeing a particular client together, making use of their own particular skills. With any co-working relationship one is considering the particular age, gender, culture and personal style of one's colleague, and considering how one can operate most effectively together as a therapeutic team.

A 14-year-old Bengali girl was reluctant to get out of bed in the morning, and was missing a great deal of school. She remained virtually monosyllabic in family interviews, and so a series of individual sessions was arranged for her in school, with an English female therapist and a Bengali female interpreter. During these sessions the girl was able to discuss a number of anxieties about growing up, and appeared in particular to appreciate the perspective offered in the interviews by the interpreter, who was closer to her own age and who had lived through many of the difficulties she described. The interpreter was encouraged by the therapist to communicate about her own experiences when growing up, and not stick strictly to her interpreting role.

Emotions

It is interesting that in Raval's study (1996) there is a complaint from therapists about a loss of emotional effect when working through an interpreter, mirrored by a comment from the interpreter interviewed in the study that she was on the receiving end of the 'emotional impact' from client families, rather than the therapist. What is going on here? The interpreter can sense the emotional impact of what the service user is experiencing, and some of this is lost to the therapist. This can have an advantage in protecting the therapist to think things through, but it may also result in the therapist not being fully in touch with the emotional experience of the service user.

Papadopoulos and Hildebrand (1997) describe the way in which the therapist who did not know their clients' language could maintain a more systemic role, keeping in mind the whole family system, rather than getting very involved in the individual's narrative. Similarly, I have at times been very grateful for the way in which interpreters have borne the brunt of client families' emotions, which I have found difficult to manage even in their muted form.

A four-year-old boy was referred because of the traumatic effects of a dispute with neighbours. The father of the child came to the centre on his own, then proceeded to recount at great length the whole story of this dispute, going back several years. In the course of telling his story through our young male locum interpreter, he made a powerful emotional connection with this young man. It was to him that he was communicating his distress, and even though the father appeared to understand the limitations of the interpreter's role, it was still to the interpreter that he seemed to look for aid and solace, asking at the end of the interview for his telephone number, rather than my (the therapist's). I had little doubt afterwards that it was the interpreter bearing this emotional weight that gave me the freedom to think, so that I was able to see the problem as most effectively dealt with at the level of a community intervention by the local housing officer, rather than being drawn into a therapeutic relationship, which would most likely have been unproductive due to the problem residing in the family's external relationships.

While training can help, interpreters will need to have a certain amount of resilience to weather such experiences; this young man needed some time to de-brief after this interview, to make sense of what had happened to him. Sometimes therapists will need to intervene, sharing more of the load by insisting that clients' communications are briefer and translated at shorter intervals, but intense emotional expression is by its nature not always amenable to such re-arrangement. As one colleague pointed out, it may be important for a client to tell his story in an uninterrupted way to another person, and this need not be the clinician.

In communications going the other way it is not my experience that the emotional effects are blunted by going through a third person. On the contrary it is my view that they can sometimes be amplified by the repetition involved in translation. Usually some family members will understand English easily and others will understand the odd word. With non-verbal gestures and expressions they will often get the gist of what I am communicating first time round, with the interpreter's version then adding weight and emphasis by going over the same ground in a different language.

Sometimes however a communication from the therapist will be viewed as far more emotionally loaded by the interpreter than the therapist. In such circumstances it may be necessary to pause and 're-group'.

I had been working for several years with a Bangladeshi family with two children with learning difficulties, whose behaviour could be difficult for the parents to manage. A 'parent advisor' had acted throughout that time as interpreter during interviews, also taking on other roles in helping the family over this time. After some months of gradually extending the period of time between interviews, and the intensity of the problems lessening, I thought the time had come to start talking about ending my contact, and attempted to ask, via the parent advisor, about the parents' views about this. I was somewhat bemused when instead of asking this question, the parent advisor got involved in talking with the parents some more about the remaining areas of difficulty. When I asked her about this she told me that she felt the family would be 'too upset' if I started talking about ending my contact at this time. The idea was at that time simply untranslatable. At the next interview when I raised the matter again, however, my ending was accepted with resignation by all concerned, evidently having been discussed by the parent advisor with the family in the interim.

I had again here committed the cardinal error of treating my colleague like a messenger, with no thoughts and feelings of her own. Apart from her ideas about the impact of my ending on the family, she would also have had feelings of her own about my ending my co-working relationship with her, leaving her to continue unsupported with a case that she would have much greater difficulty in closing, given the more extensive nature of her role. And here was I expecting her to translate these words without any prior discussion with her about their impact on her and on the family.

One way in which clinicians can shorten the emotional distance between themselves and their clients while using an interpreter is to address their clients directly ('you should do this'), rather than through the interpreter in the third person ('she should do this'). This is recommended as good practice by Shackman (1984) and by Freed (1988). Another way is to make use of seating positions, placing the interpreter so that the client is facing the clinician – Shackman (1984) indicates that common practice in Australia when she wrote her book was for interpreters to sit behind the clients. Such working methods would clearly increase the intensity of the interaction between client and clinician, but this would be at the expense of making therapeutic use of the knowledge and personality of the interpreter, and his/her relationship with the client. Such an understanding of interpretation makes it more an art than a science or as Geertz (1983) put it, 'rather closer to what a critic does to illumine a poem than what an astronomer does to account for a star'.

Getting on the same wavelength

Of course it is only with interpreters that one is working alongside regularly that one can develop such mutual knowledge and working practices over the course of time. Like any other form of co-working, initially there will be more of a need for planning time before interviews with clients, in which some of these mutual beliefs and working practices can be explored. Both therapist and interpreter will need to orientate themselves to one another, in order to maximise the effectiveness of their collaboration. Before commencing an interview with a family with an adolescent girl where there are concerns about her eating, for example, it is likely to be helpful to explore in a pre-planning session ideas about what such behaviour may mean, as well as what is likely to be helpful in overcoming such difficulties.

There will be times of course in which interpreters, in attempting to bring about greater understanding between the two parties, will cause misunderstanding. Farooq et al (1997) checked on the accuracy of one Mirpuri speaking interpreter by a Mirpuri speaking psychiatrist scrutinizing the audiotapes of the interpreter's interviews, in which she interpreted between Mirpuri speaking patients and an English psychiatrist. A number of 'common errors' were noted, such as omission (where a message was deleted), condensation (where lengthy responses were simplified), and 'subtle changes' in the way questions were asked. Many of these 'errors' can be understood as the interpreter making a judgement about what the clinician's intention is in asking certain questions (to make a psychiatric diagnosis), and selecting and extrapolating from what is being said accordingly. For example one exchange is quoted as follows:

PSYCHIATRIST: Do you feel happy or sad in your spirits?
PATIENT: If I am not unhappy or sad . . . (pause) . . . then I am happy
INTERPRETER: (without interpreting this response) You feel sad now?
PATIENT: Yes
INTERPRETER: She is unhappy

One way of making sense of this interchange is that the interpreter is working on an assumption about what information the psychiatrist is interested in, and tailoring how she interprets accordingly. Hence she ignores the reference to happy feelings in the patient's communication, focusing instead on the symptoms that she supposes the psychiatrist is seeking to identify. A 'brief solution' clinician (de Shazer, 1988) would be more interested in eliciting positive talk from clients, identifying 'exceptions' where clients have achieved some mastery over their problems. If the interpreter had been working with such a clinician and if she had been familiar with this way of working, she might have picked up on what the patient initially said differently, highlighting the statement about happiness rather than drawing forth more communication about the unhappiness.

Two into three won't go

Rachel Tribe (1991) mentions that in support groups run for interpreters an issue raised was the way in which someone is always 'left out' in the interpreting triangle. Both the therapist and the client will have periods of waiting for the others to finish speaking, not understanding what is being said. This experience can be extremely uncomfortable: Freed (1988) describes an interpreter giving 'painfully brief' translations of her interviewee's long answers.

The 'pain' here is presumably caused to the interviewer because she is feeling excluded from a significant part of her interviewee's communications, which is causing her frustration and resentment. The context she describes (conducting interviews in a foreign country) made it difficult for her to make sense of her interpreter's brevity, and to find a more satisfactory form of collaboration. Such feelings will be less likely to arise where clinicians and interpreters have developed a relationship of mutual trust over a period of time, but even with such a relationship there will be times when a clinician will need to ask about such discrepancies. Clients too at times will feel unsure that their communications have been properly interpreted (many bring their own unofficial interpreters in the form of family friends or relatives to begin with). Clients should also be encouraged to question the clinician or interpreter, and check that the interpreter or clinician has accurately understood their concerns.

Power, professionalism and the place of training

I suspect some of the pain described above is down to the interviewer feeling powerless, not a comfortable position for professionals who are used to feeling in charge of the interviews they are conducting. Freed's (1988) solution to such difficulties involves the training of interpreters, and for other workers to view interpreters as fellow professionals, rather than subordinates. She adds that interpreters need a sense of participation and accomplishment, for data to be assembled with reasonable accuracy.

In any working partnership a sense of both parties being valued and appreciated for their contribution will add to the cohesion of the partnership, and limit the potential for mutual distrust and competitiveness. Training and professionalisation of interpreters is one concrete way in which organisations can show that these workers are valued. It could go some way to decrease the types of problems described that can arise in the work (Block, 1996; Raval, 1996). Westermeyer (1990) suggests that psychiatric interpreters should be familiar with (and hence need training in): medical, psychiatric, psychological and social terminology; techniques of interviewing; the importance of non-verbal communication; normal and abnormal psychology; therapies used in psychiatric care; cultural influences on mental status examination; and methods of asking about matters that do not come up in ordinary communication, like hallucinations and sexual problems. As Shackman (1984) argued, the employment of interpreters should be viewed as a 'step towards appropriate provision, rather than the solution', this being the training and employment of ethnic minority staff for more traditional, highly valued professions. Miller and Krause (1995) describe one model for the creation and training of such staff.

However, clinicians also need training in being able to work with interpreters. One example of a useful joint training exercise encouraging self-reflexivity in clinicians and interpreters has been to study videotapes of interviews, with the interpreter re-interpreting back into English his interpretations of the clinician's utterances. One such revision exercise revealed striking differences, particularly for longer utterances, with the interpreter placing more emphasis on the parts of the clinician's communications that meant more for him. Discussion of such differences led to the development of a more self-conscious practice, with more checking out of one another's meaning during interviews.

Another way in which the power imbalance can be addressed is by the therapist's attitude and demeanour towards the interpreter during interviews. The interpreter quoted above (p. 144) felt used, in a way that did not allow for any degree of mutuality in the work. A practice in which interpreters' knowledge and expertise is included in the therapeutic process, being accorded due respect as a perspective that may have particular usefulness because of the interpreters' shared experience with clients, would carry a very different message about the status accorded to each party. This interaction between the co-workers carries with it an important communication to clients about the clinician's intention to respect other perspectives, and not to impose his/her values and ways of seeing things.

An alternative model: making meaning together

Such a practice rests upon a very different model of communication from the 'post office' model described above; communication is 'lived in' rather than something we stand outside and make use of (Pearce, 1989). Rather than a means by which 'internal' states are expressed and 'objective' facts represented, communication is seen as the process by which we construct together a shared way of understanding such states and facts. Interpreters, rather than being seen as the impersonal agents of clinicians (avoiding at all costs contaminating the purity of the clinician's communication), become a vital part of the construction of a shared meaning, whose own history and personhood are a vital part. Rather than attempting to 'filter out' this personhood, its impact upon the ongoing work is recognised, appreciated and embraced as something that will enrich and enhance this work.

Pearce (1989) used the term 'cosmopolitan communication' to describe a style of communication that in no way assumes the superiority of our own ways of making meaning, based on the premise that we have all been shaped by the particularities of our own culture and historical experience, which has given us all a different view of reality, a different way of describing it, of making sense of it. He points out that major differences exist even within groups, that we often underestimate the 'otherness' of other people, from whom we are 'separated by the use of a common language'.

According to such a model good practice in working alongside interpreters with clients with a different language is no different in essence from good practice in working with clients who share the same language; in the way that nothing is taken for granted about each individual's unique way of seeing the world, their values or their use of language, and each person's world-view is accorded equal status with our own. If anything such a practice is easier to maintain with clients who speak a different language, as we are far less likely to make assumptions about what is meant. It comes far more naturally to ask a client from rural Sylhet in Bangladesh via an interpreter what they mean when they use words like 'independence' or 'honour', than it does for a client sharing a common language with us, though differences may be just as great. Also discussing openly with one's interpreter the words he/she is using in translating such concepts is in the spirit of such 'cosmopolitan communication': conveying an appreciation of the different ways in which experience is understood; adding to the depth and complexity of the work undertaken; and allowing clients more of a choice of possible meanings to draw from, in thinking about their lives.

Acknowledgements

My thanks to my colleagues at the Emanuel Miller Centre for their many contributions towards the development of the ideas in this chapter, and in particular to the interpreters Pheyara Nizam and Nurul Huque whose sensitivity and thoughtfulness in our work together has been an inspiration.

References

Amato, R. (1992) 'One of the Titans'. In V. O'Sullivan (ed.), *The Oxford Book of New Zealand Short Stories*. Auckland: Oxford University Press.

Block, E. (1996) 'Ideas about cultural difference in a multidisciplinary team'. Unpublished MSc Thesis, Tavistock Clinic.

de Shazer, S. (1988) *Clues: Investigating Solutions in Brief Therapy*. New York: Norton.

Farooq, S., Fear, C. and Oyebode, F. (1997) 'An investigation of the adequacy of psychiatric interviews conducted through an interpreter'. *Psychiatric Bulletin*, 21: 209–213.

Freed, A. (1988) 'Interviewing through an interpreter'. *Social Work*, 33: 315–319.

Geertz, C. (1983) *Local Knowledge*. New York: Basic Books.

Harvey, M. (1984) 'Family therapy with deaf persons: the systemic utilisation of an interpreter'. *Family Process*, 23: 205–213.

Miller, A. and Krause, B. (1995) 'Culture and family therapy'. In S. Fernando (ed.), *Mental Health in a Multi Ethnic Society: A Multidisciplinary Handbook*. London: Routledge.

Miller, G. (1986) 'What We Say and What We Mean'. *New York Times Book Review*, Jan. 26: p. 37.

Minuchin, S. and Fishman, C. (1981) *Family Therapy Techniques*. Cambridge: Harvard University Press.

Pearce, W. Barnett (1989) *Communication and the Human Condition*. Carbondale, IL: Southern Illinois University Press.

Papadopoulos, R. and Hildebrand, J. (1997) 'Is home where the heart is? Narratives of oppositional discourses in refugee families'. In R. Papadopoulos and J. Byng-Hall (eds), *Multiple Voices: Narrative in Systemic Family Psychotherapy*. London: Duckworth.

Raval, H. (1996) 'A systemic perspective on working with interpreters'. *Clinical Child Psychology and Psychiatry*, 1: 29–43.

Rennie, S. (1998) *Interpreting and Access to Public Services*. Bradford: Sequals.

Shackman, J. (1984) *The Right to be Understood: A Handbook on Working with, Employing, and Training Community Interpreters*. Cambridge: National Extension College.

Tribe, R. (1991) 'Bi-cultural workers – bridging the gap or damming the flow?'. Paper presented at the II International Conference of Centres, Institutions and Individuals concerned with the care of victims of violence, health, political repression and human rights. Santiago, Chile.

Westermeyer, J. (1990) 'Working with an interpreter in psychiatric assessment and treatment'. *The Journal of Nervous and Mental Disease*, 178: 745–749.

Wittgenstein, L. (1953) *Philosophical Investigations*. Oxford: Blackwell.

Chapter 10

The role of the interpreter in child mental health: the changing landscape

Rosemary Loshak

In the early 1980s, changing patterns of immigration resulted in a rapid increase in the Bangladeshi population of East London as wives and children came from Bangladesh to join their husbands in an established though small and mostly male community, which had existed in the area for 20 to 30 years. The massive demographic changes that followed had consequences for the organisation and delivery of services in health, education and social services with each agency struggling to find its own response to the challenges posed by differences of language and culture. Today over 60 per cent of the school age population in the area are of Bangladeshi origin. Although for these second generation immigrants their first language is now English, for their parents and for those children newly arrived from Bangladesh their first language remains Sylheti. The provision of an effective and sensitive child mental health service to this population has presented professionals and their managers with the need to examine their practice and adapt to rapidly changing needs. The efforts of a multi-disciplinary team to develop its work with families across this linguistic divide are the subject of this chapter.

An early research initiative examined parental perceptions of the service among Bangladeshi families (Hillier et al, 1994). In all areas of health care it is increasingly understood that mutual sharing and understanding of treatment goals between patient and therapist facilitates compliance with treatment and hence positive outcome. This study, examining a small sample of families referred to the service, supported this view noting that good communication, leading to a shared understanding of the problems, led to parental satisfaction and was correlated with positive outcomes. A process that empowers parents rather than undermining them is likely to be beneficial for the child.

Immigrants inevitably bring with them, as well as excitement, energy and hope for the future, experiences of loss and separation, of divided families, and divided loyalties. Their high expectations of their new life in Britain are often disappointed as they encounter poor housing conditions and relative poverty in the face of unheard-of affluence. They bring different religious beliefs that will support their sense of identity in an often-hostile environment but also a set of beliefs and attitudes about the organisation of British society that are rooted in an experience of colonial power and rural poverty. Previous experiences of authority internalised in a very different cultural environment will be transferred into and shape this new relationship. Rack (1982) has described the prevalent experience of authority among rural peasant populations as harsh, punitive and often corrupt. Figures of authority are seen, not as benign and potentially helpful but as liable to exploit the individual and therefore to be circumvented. Thus when a concerned teacher enlists the help of a Sylheti speaking playground assistant to encourage a parent to seek help from Social Services, the message conveyed may be quite different from that intended and cast blame on the parent for bringing shame on the community by not managing her children without outside intervention.

Families will invariably experience overt racism on the streets and indirect racism within the public institutions on which they are heavily dependent, such as schools and hospitals, as these slowly become more responsive to the new population. All of these factors will shape and determine the nature of their encounter with professionals, still generally white, who have their own set of values, beliefs and attitudes. The lack of familiarity with helping agencies such as a child mental health team, unknown in rural Bangladesh, may lead to inappropriate expectations.

All of these factors enter into the dialogue between therapists and families so that an interpreter needs not only good linguistic skills but also an awareness of these processes as they operate within themselves and in all the parties in the room so that families can feel understood and accepted. This chapter sets out to explore this interaction through presenting case material and to describe the process of recruiting and integrating a Sylheti speaking interpreter into a child mental health team. Identifying details have been changed to protect confidentiality.

The experience of all those involved in the following encounter may illustrate the potential for dissatisfaction that exists where there is inadequate provision and preparation. Mujid was a 15-year-old boy. His social worker referred him to the child mental health service for a psychiatric assessment pending a court appearance. She was concerned about violence in the family and believed Mujid might be beaten at home. The family was invited to attend and a Sylheti speaking interpreter was booked from a hospital-wide advocacy service. The family arrived late having got lost in the hospital. The hospital interpreter also arrived late, rushing from another busy outpatient clinic. There was little opportunity for briefing her. The therapists began by asking the family if they understood why they were there. As the hospital interpreter conveyed this question Mr Ali, Mujid's father, began to talk animatedly to her, avoiding eye contact with the therapists; he explained that Mujid was a good boy, and had not committed the offence. The hospital interpreter in an advocacy role, conveyed his response and the therapists heard her as pleading the case for the boy's innocence. They were unable to include the mother, Mrs Begum, who might have known more about Mujid's behaviour and they wondered about communication within the family. Mr Ali had recently returned from Bangladesh and seemed not to have been told of Mujid's behaviour in his absence. The therapists' anxiety mounted as they struggled to open up communication. They began to feel persecuting, unable to intervene, out of control of the interview. Questions directed at the whole family to encourage reflection were directed by the hospital interpreter at Mujid and became transformed into blaming, persecutory attacks, reinforcing his withdrawal. The hospital interpreter, unable to tolerate the discomfort of the ensuing silence, pressed him to reply, joining with the parents, while the therapists felt increasingly paralysed by frustration and impotence.

Such experiences leave all parties at best dissatisfied and probably bitter and demoralised. Mujid and his family had yet another experience of not being understood. They may see the encounter as irrelevant and time-wasting or as arbitrary and persecuting, reinforcing an already paranoid view of a hostile world. The hospital interpreter may leave feeling no one is pleased with her efforts and may be reluctant to return to this team where the work is so difficult. The therapists may experience a deep unhappiness that their drive toward understanding and helping has had such an obviously unsatisfactory outcome. There has been no explanation of the purpose of the meeting and expected outcomes. The hospital interpreter and therapists are unclear about their respective roles and functions and this confusion has interfered with the process of the interview.

For this family the service was probably experienced as irrelevant, confusing and of little positive value. One might wonder whether the organisation, in addressing the problems of language difference through an under-resourced interpreting service trying to cover the whole hospital, is simply providing a short-term solution to a situation which is much more complex.

Both for the organisation and the individual, interpreting, rather than bridging a gap between professionals in institutions and the immigrant communities they are trying to serve, can function to maintain a comfortable distance protecting the professional and his/her institution from the unbearable pain of exclusion, alienation and marginalisation which immigrant families are facing. If immigrant communities are to have adequate access to specialist services such as child mental health they need much more than accurate linguistic interpretation. They need information about the service and encouragement to attend. They need friendly reception staff and the possibility of telephone contact in their own language. They need reassurance about confidentiality and explanation of roles and function. Above all they need to make emotional contact with professionals who can move freely and comfortably across cultural boundaries themselves and bear to listen to painful experiences. The interpreter's own skills, knowledge and capacity for empathy are crucial to such contact being effective.

Experience in adult services in Bradford points to the use of a job description that more accurately reflects the complexity of the work and the extent to which the responsibility for the encounter is shared between therapist and interpreter. Following their example we have used the title of bilingual communications assistant or bilingual worker (Bavington, 1992).

A child mental health team in context

The service provided by a child mental health team is determined and influenced by agencies and factors external to the team itself as well as by its own shared values and professional ethos. Some consideration of these is necessary to an understanding of the nature of the clinical encounter.

While the 1989 Children Act requires that local authorities have regard to the race, and ethnicity of children and their families in providing services for them, the need for culturally appropriate provision in the health service is based in standards of good practice rather than in statute with the result that staffing changes and the recruitment of interpreters may be slow. A national review of child mental health services commented that 'the matching of provision to local needs has hardly begun' but made no explicit mention of the ethnicity of staff as an important factor (Kurtz et al, 1994).

When a service such as child mental health operates under tight financial restraints with many competing claims for resources, provision to meet the language needs of minority groups may come low in the list of priorities. While Social Services and Education departments have made use of funding through the Race Relations Act to recruit ethnic minority staff and increasingly employ a multicultural workforce, this has not been available in health trusts. A health based child mental health team may in consequence, while encompassing a diversity of experience, theoretical approach and disciplines, remain limited in its awareness of issues of race, language and cultural difference. Professionals may be mostly white and distanced from local culture.

In East London while there are small communities of Somali, Vietnamese, Chinese and Pakistani peoples (for whom interpreting provision and access to services remains severely limited) the largest minority group are of Bangladeshi origin, forming 35 per cent of the population. This contrasts with Inner London as a whole where the population is 58 per cent white and 7.1 per cent Bangladeshi. With the rapid growth in this community Social Services and Education have responded by recruiting and training Bangladeshi staff. There are substantial numbers of Bengali or Sylheti speaking social workers including team managers and above. Most schools employ Bangladeshi classroom assistants, playground helpers and special needs assistants. Community health settings include Sylheti speaking link-workers or interpreters, while some more specialist settings employ parent advisers to work directly with families. There is a small but growing professional workforce of psychologists, counsellors, teachers and educational psychologists.

Patterns of immigration, changing over time, bring particular difficulties and have an impact on services. An outline of these changes is necessary to an understanding of the problems faced by families and by services today.

The early migrants were men now in their sixties coming as seamen as a result of long established colonial trade with the jute producing areas of Bengal. In the 1970s and early 1980s, women and children joined their husbands here but there was often a considerable age-gap between husband and wife and fathers were virtual strangers to their children born in Bangladesh. Today many of these young women have become widows bringing up large families of young children alone, often without the support of an extended family and with little command of English. Such situations frequently arouse concern in other agencies resulting in referral to a child mental health team but the difficulties involved for these families in getting to the clinic may seem overwhelming. Children often have a number of different appointments with a number of different health professionals on various sites. To bring small children by public transport is a daunting task.

Literacy levels remain low as women in particular may have had only a few years' formal education. Fluency in English is correspondingly low with 12 per cent of fathers and 45 per cent of mothers speaking no English at all (Tomlinson and Hutchison, 1991). Printed information about the child mental health service may not be read or understood and appointment letters may be wrongly translated or ignored by English speaking children translating for their parents!

Immigrants may bring with them high expectations of health care but limited understanding of treatment approaches in western medical care. The stigma of mental illness, or any behaviour that can bring shame on the family and thus reduce other family members' chances of success in life, is acute and can result in families viewing first appointments with dread. Families do not know what to expect when they arrive at a clinic and few white professionals feel confident to give a basic greeting in Bengali, to put a family at ease.

Nevertheless, the community is far from homogeneous and is in a state of constant change, adjustment and growth. The extended family, even when divided between two continents, can remain a force for cohesion and emotional support. The community has a vitality and energy reflected in its political life, cultural and religious celebrations, and abundance of thriving social groups. A striking feature is the number of young people, second-generation immigrants, now graduating from university with a strong commitment to serve the community to which they belong.

A child mental health team has to be open and alive to all aspects of these experiences, not merely to the pathology, if it is to begin to provide an appropriate service. It has to retain its integrity and professional values while being sufficiently permeable to respond sensitively to the diversity of the community which it serves. The extent to which bilingualism can become a fully incorporated aspect of team life, and bilingual workers integrated into the organisational structure, may reflect the team's capacity for openness. Recruitment of a bilingual worker to assist with all aspects of communication with Bangladeshi families has been a significant first step.

Recruitment of a bilingual worker

In 1990 the service secured resources to employ a Bangladeshi worker part-time as a bilingual communications assistant providing interpreting over three geographically separate sites. The team set aside time for some preparatory work before the appointment. This involved circulating already published material about working with interpreters, which helped raise some important questions in a team discussion (Shackman, 1984).

In the absence at that time of established training or career structures for interpreters the team felt it was important to be clear about the personal characteristics and experience required. To employ someone with professional qualifications, e.g. in medicine or teaching, seemed an inappropriate step likely to lead to both misunderstandings about role and to resentments. An interest in mental health and some experience with children or families were the selection criteria and personal qualities were given considerable weight at interview. A simple role-play with a Sylheti speaker served to demonstrate fluency in Sylheti at interview.

In order to provide maximum access for families full-time employment of bilingual workers is essential. The post (and then a further post) have been advertised and recruited on a part-time basis and have attracted high quality staff. However in the long term a part-time post is inadequate to service needs, does not bring sufficient job satisfaction and may impede career development. A full-time appointment with prospects of advancement is more likely to attract applicants with the necessary commitment, calibre and maturity while a service willing to invest in and prepare adequately for its own dedicated worker will be more likely to attract those with the necessary interest and sensitivity for work in mental health (Barnett, 1989).

While there was a shared hope that the worker would have many functions in addition to interpretation, such as cultural adviser to the team, educator for trainees, consultant on appropriate treatment methods, there were also many unanswered questions about the extent to which the worker might work on their own, or be seen as co-therapist. With no established professional structure for interpreters the team had to consider the need for support and supervision and how this might be provided. There were anxieties about the emotional impact of the work on a team member who might be quite isolated as well as more practical concerns about managing the booking of time.

The discussion allowed every team member to be involved in the process and take responsibility for making the appointment work. Slowly a shared view emerged that the post could develop over time as the worker gained confidence and experience, leading to opportunities for training and advancement.

With the appointment of one, then two part-time bilingual workers as members of two teams, some previously unconsidered factors have emerged. The bilingual worker is likely to be a member of the local community and to feel more vulnerable to direct personal questions or attempts by families to contact him or her outside the clinic. He or she is also likely to be one of the lowest paid staff in the team and to identify closely with families' experiences of financial hardship. All teams are vulnerable under stress to resentment and envy arising from inequalities of salary and status but the way in which such feelings may affect an unqualified worker from a minority group needs to be held in mind. The service took pains from the outset to ensure that bilingual workers were fully integrated team members, expected to attend team meetings and training events and to have regular supervision despite this reducing available interpreting time. The team felt strongly that the bilingual worker had a particular role in these contexts in bringing a transcultural perspective to all the team's thinking. They also recognised the emotional strain of seeing distressed clients without respite. Such matters need to be negotiated with and supported by sympathetic managers.

The child mental health team includes not only different professions but also staff at different levels of experience using different theoretical models in their work. The team bilingual worker moves constantly between them all needing to be sure of him or herself yet sufficiently open to different ways of working. He or she will need to become conversant with the various theoretical approaches and able to work comfortably with them all.

With a worker in post the team was later able to monitor and audit its way of working. The bilingual worker felt interviews progressed more satisfactorily when she was allowed some flexibility to clarify things for the family, to intervene when there were gaps or difficulties in the communication and to interpret the emotional atmosphere of the session. Professionals commented on feeling more distant from the process and being aware of a stronger therapeutic alliance forming between the family and the bilingual worker.

The child's experience

My first language:
A relief, a comfortable secret helping me, hindering me,
making me a stranger.
My second language:
Powerful.
Two strange languages inside my head.
    Juan Berganinos Fuentes – aged 15, Pimlico School, 1981
                    (Council for Racial Equality 1996)

What does it mean to be a Bangladeshi child coming for the first time to a child mental health clinic? 5-year-old Lipi was electively mute. Referred by her school she spoke only within the confines of her immediate family. Her mother did not need an interpreter, her English was fluent. During the first interview in which the team bilingual assistant remained present Lipi herself did not speak at all, ignored the white therapist but made repeated tentative efforts to engage the bilingual worker in silent communication by touching, looking and smiling. Slowly she became more relaxed, engaged in play and at later sessions began to speak directly to the therapist. Lipi was able to explore an unfamiliar setting at her own pace and under the watchful and encouraging eye of another maternal figure, that of the bilingual worker. The white therapist was free to focus on

Lipi's mother's anxieties. Perhaps for Lipi and her mother the experience was of feeling secure in the presence of a familiar figure of their own culture.

More frequently a child has to manage her anxiety in an unfamiliar setting, while having at the same time to attune to the two languages being used. The bilingual child has to function as his own interpreter throughout the session and his needs may be overlooked. The bilingual worker is best placed to check the child's understanding and to give the child a voice in his own language. The child may then have the rare experience of a partnership between thinking adults of different races and cultures, using different languages but nevertheless between them able to contain his anxieties and find a form of expression for them which all can understand.

For 8-year-old Shipu this proved salutary. When the therapist addressed him directly knowing his English to be good he smiled charmingly but spoke in Bengali. As the therapist was quietly informed by her bilingual colleague that he was directing obscenities at her and at his mother he became openly angry. As his anger gave way to distress a real discussion of his difficulties could take place. An interpreter unfamiliar with the work and without a safe relationship with a therapist might feel less than comfortable in interpreting such language or might react unhelpfully by reprimanding him.

Children born in Bangladesh, having emigrated with their families, quickly acquire basic language skills. However these may deter rather than assist communication as the professional assumes a level of understanding while the child continues to think in Bengali, and to struggle beneath the surface in a sea of confusion, with little real comprehension. Ayres (1994) has distinguished the adaptive part of the child making links with the new culture, and the infant part in touch with difficult feelings which we so easily fail to recognise.

A meeting with 11-year-old Rumena and her family describes this process. After only 2 years in Britain, Rumena was not coping with the move to secondary school. Her teachers complained of poor concentration and wondered if she had learning difficulties. Attempts by the therapist to talk to her directly seemed to paralyse her. Interpretation into Sylheti made little headway, she remained silent and withdrawn. Her mother was equally reticent and her father repeatedly spoke for his wife as well. Rumena's 15-year-old sister took responsibility for explaining Rumena's problems and translating for her father. Only when the bilingual worker gently insisted that she would interpret for everyone could a story slowly emerge of a mother who had a psychiatric illness, of Rumena being cared for by her grandparents now left behind in Bangladesh and of her older sister taking on a parenting role. The bilingual worker's calm assertion of her own authority and her knowledge of the character of village life in rural Sylhet contained the therapist's feelings of anxiety and confusion. She was enabled to reflect on these and with the family begin to understand Rumena's loss of much-loved grandparents and her confusion on moving from the village to an urban environment. As these became real to the therapist, Rumena's regression to infantile behaviour became understandable and the parents were helped to acknowledge her feelings and support her emotionally.

An older child may need the bilingual worker to interpret not only words but also customs and rules governing family behaviour.

Shahel, aged 12, attended with his father. The therapist suggested he talk directly to his father about his schoolwork, his ambitions and interests, and further that he ask his father to tell him about his own childhood in Bangladesh. The bilingual worker explained to the therapist that it was unacceptable for Shahel to ask these questions unless his father raised them first.

Together the workers can then explore possibilities of changing this pattern and improving communication and understanding within this family. The bilingual worker has indicated important cultural differences in parental behaviour and introduced the parents' perspective, thus shedding light on the difficulty and reducing the therapist's frustration and misunderstanding.

Understanding parental concerns

Most parents will come to a first appointment in a child mental heath service with considerable apprehension; anxiety about their child's well being, feelings of failure as parents, and a sense of shame at involvement with psychiatric services. For immigrant families such feelings are further reinforced by the lack of familiarity with the service, by the loss of containing helpful parental figures resulting from immigration, and by the experiences of racism, poverty, and unemployment. It is no easy task for professionals to remain alert to such feelings and to the part they play in deciding whether or not a family engages in treatment. A few minutes at the beginning of a first interview when the bilingual assistant talks about the setting and puts the family at ease assuring them of confidentiality, can do much to overcome such anxieties and aid the process of engagement. A bilingual worker, sure of her own place in the professional team, acts as a role model giving a powerful message to parents and children that they too will be treated with respect, can ask questions and proceed at their own pace.

The personal qualities of the bilingual worker, his or her interpreting style, and the relationship with the therapist are all of crucial importance.

Shamina, a 15-year-old girl, presented in an emergency with hysterical fits. Her parents conveyed very powerfully their anxiety and fear. They were frightened for her health and of the consequences of what they perceived to be a serious mental illness with its attached shame and stigma. Shamina's mother, Johura, sat seemingly talking to herself and unreachable. An interpreter from the hospital interpreting service was unable to allay the fears that Johura could only manage by constant prayer. Later we learned that this interpreter was known personally to these parents, who were made more anxious and fearful that news of their daughter's condition would be spread around the community. Such intense and paranoid anxiety as these parents expressed cannot be ignored but requires patient and systematic response by an empathic worker, who is attuned to community attitudes and cultural beliefs about mental illness but with an optimism based on experience of things getting better.

The relationship established between parents and therapist may mirror that existing between therapist and bilingual worker. Where a worker assumes an air of deference towards his or her therapist colleague, creating a setting in which therapists are seen as experts, the family may respond with compliance and make frequent expressions of gratitude and politeness. However, families also present with frustration and hostility, sometimes expressed in the children's behaviour or hidden behind compliant smiles. A bilingual worker experienced in mental health who is able to tolerate silence and bear some of the negative projections will enable the therapist to make interpretations which allow true feelings to be vented. Yet it requires considerable trust to translate hostile comments directed at the therapist or abusive or critical remarks directed at the interpreter herself. Dilwar, father of Shamina, implied that the therapist was not doing all she might to help his daughter. As the bilingual worker was able to bear and to convey his impatience and frustration, she and the therapist were able to acknowledge the rage and impotence he was feeling and enable him to understand his own contribution to his daughter's difficulties.

These parents, presenting in crisis, saw four different interpreters before regular work with the team bilingual worker could be established. At their third visit a hospital interpreter was present, a quiet and courteous older man who clearly evoked in Johura memories of her own father whom she now told us had died some years earlier. He had been an important internal figure who had become unavailable to her and was now revived in her mind. At their next visit however a different interpreter arrived and this important link was lost. These parents were not able to entrust their daughter to the therapist for regular individual sessions until their anxieties could be contained by the consistent attendance of the team bilingual worker at family meetings.

That the interpreter has this important role in providing containment may be difficult for professionals to acknowledge and allow.

Shahel's mother arrived heavily pregnant and unwell; the team bilingual worker was encouraged to attend to her complaints, enabling her to tell an empathic listener the extent to which she felt alone with the responsibility for her children's welfare, unsupported by a much older, emotionally distant husband. She became more thoughtful, reflecting on her situation, recognising that her anxieties about Shahel were inappropriate to his actual behaviour. She began to speak with greater assurance, using English to the therapist. The trust between the therapist and her bilingual colleague, and the therapist's capacity to remain relatively uninvolved functioned for this woman as a container of her disturbance, giving space for her own thoughts to develop.

Where a therapist is able to tolerate her own inactivity, allowing a family to be contained and understood by the bilingual worker in their own language, he/she is free to observe, to reflect on his/her own feelings and to think more creatively about what might be happening in the encounter. As parents feel confident to ask questions they find their own capacity for thought. Thoughts can be exchanged and new shared understandings emerge. However the three-person encounter of parent, therapist, and interpreter is potentially problematic when feelings of exclusion become overwhelming. Where these are contained by a relationship developed over time between therapist and bilingual worker, a space is opened up for creative thinking between all three participants.

Relationships with the team

The bilingual worker, lacking professional status, has to value her own contribution and be valued by her colleagues. There are times when families bring so much despair and hopelessness that no-one can feel positive about what has been achieved. The bilingual worker needs to become able to recognise this and to distinguish those occasions when it is the conduct of the interview, for which she shares responsibility, that has led to feelings of failure.

For example, in a meeting with two parents and a family therapist the bilingual worker began to feel excluded, redundant and useless. Reflecting on this she realised that the male therapist was engaged in an interesting conversation with Mr Hussein, the child's father, while the mother was being ignored. Being sufficiently confident of her own role and relationship with this more senior team member, she was able to interrupt him and point out what was happening for the benefit of all concerned.

At times there may be two therapists in addition to the bilingual worker seeing a family and the practice of taking a break for therapists to think and formulate may be employed. It is worth considering the part of the bilingual worker in this. If he/she remains with the family, not included in this thinking process, he/she may be left feeling undermined and at a loss to understand the treatment plans he/she is supposed to convey to the family. He/she can become identified with the family's feelings of alienation and marginalisation. The family may receive a message that Bangladeshi workers are not valued and respected, which may have a direct impact on their own self-esteem.

In a first meeting with a family there are many tasks such as clarifying the role of the agency, conveying the meaning of confidentiality, putting a family at ease. Some therapists will want to engage the family themselves at this stage, seeing this early discussion as integral to the whole encounter. Others will more readily give up these tasks in part to the bilingual worker who can use his/her own experience and knowledge of families' initial responses and convey the quality of the exchange to the therapist in a general way. The bilingual worker needs to be flexible in his/her response to different therapists but also needs to demand some freedom for him/herself in determining how to conduct these early stages of the encounter.

As a session progresses a family may want to repeat what has been said, perhaps for clarification, and the bilingual worker will want the space to do that without the need for interpretation while at the same time remaining sensitive to the therapist's purpose and goals. Such sharing of responsibility can only take place where there is mutual respect and where the bilingual worker is recognised as a fully integrated member of the team with his/her own unique function.

In the professional team he/she may be the only non-white, ethnic minority member. As such his/her physical presence in team meetngs, in the office and staff room is not only an ever-present resource but also brings the minority culture to life in the team. On a daily basis the team shares aspects of his/her family life, his/her traditions, his/her religious values and in so doing builds up a store of images and experience of a different culture, as well as finding connections with their own and identifying what is shared. For a team which may receive a distorted view of a minority community through a client group that includes the most disadvantaged and dysfunctional families, this picture of strong and healthy relationships provides a very necessary balance and wider perspective. At the same time his/her understanding of the experiences of immigration and racism in particular helps ensure that the team remains in touch with these factors and more sensitive in its response. The knowledge about culture and community that the team had sought to learn in formal teaching comes through knowing the person of the bilingual worker.

Future development of the role

A bilingual team member acts as a bridge to facilitate ethnic minority families' access to the service. His/her presence in the office and reception, and his/her availability to speak to families on the telephone, improves accessibility in a very immediate way. This can be extended by making the bilingual worker the first point of contact for such families either in their own home or in a school or other community base.

Some workers, some teams and some managers may prefer to maintain this fairly limited role, while others will see the post as a means of drawing able and committed individuals into the service and training them for more complex work. Bilingual workers will have varying aspirations and working styles, which may enable them to go on to further training as counsellor, family therapist or in an organisational or educational role. The model of a parent adviser has been developed elsewhere in the neighbouring boroughs in East London and could usefully be extended into child mental health, where an appropriately trained bilingual worker could offer parental support and behavioural management advice.

With increasing referrals co-therapy has decreased in the team except where the language barrier demands the presence of a bilingual worker. This can be seen as a rare opportunity for an apprentice model of learning with an increasing share of the work being given to the bilingual worker under conditions of maximum supervision and support.

Developing skills of this kind requires trust and close knowledge of the others work. It demands an openness on the part of professionals, managers and their organisations to the creative possibilities of individuals, which may be difficult to hold on to in the present climate of financial restraint and control.

The part played by interpreters in child mental health is significantly different from that in other health settings, since conveying subjective experience, affect and meaning are as important as gathering information and are essential to the therapeutic process. The complexity of the dynamics within the family and between family and workers needs to be grasped and worked with. The setting provides a unique opportunity for the development of skills and potential of individuals with commitment to the service. Such development can only help the service to become more responsive to the changing needs of the community.

References

Ayres, W. (1994) 'Foreword'. In I.A. Canino and J. Spurlock (ed.), *Culturally Diverse Children and Adolescents: Assessment, Diagnosis and Treatment*. New York: Guilford Press.

Barnett, S. (1989) 'Working with interpreters'. In D.M. Duncan (ed.), *Working with Bilingual Language Disability*. London: Chapman and Hall.

Bavington, J. (1992) 'The Bradford Experience'. In J. Kareem and R. Littlewood (eds), *Intercultural Therapy, Themes, Interpretations and Practice*. Oxford: Blackwell.

Council for Racial Equality (1996) *Roots of the Future: Ethnic Diversity in the Making of Britain*. London: HMSO.

Hillier, S., Loshak, R., Rahman, S. and Marks, F. (1994) 'An evaluation of child psychiatric services for Bangladeshi parents'. *Journal of Mental Health*, 3: 327–337.

Kurtz, Z., Thornes, R. and Wolkind, S. (1994) *Services for the Mental Health of Children and Young People in England; a National Review*. Maudsley Hospital and South Thames (West) Regional Health Authority.

Rack, P. (1982) *Race, Culture and Mental Disorder*. London: Tavistock.

Shackman, J. (1984) *The Right to be Understood: a Handbook for Working with Community Interpreters*. Cambridge: National Extension College.

Tomlinson, S. and Hutchison, S. (1991) *Bangladeshi Parents and Education in Tower Hamlets*. Lancaster: Advisory Centre for Education, University of Lancaster.

Chapter 11

Working with interpreters within services for people with learning disabilities

John Newland

Introduction

What follows is an attempt at providing a framework for clinicians using interpreters in services for people with learning disabilities (pwld). The absolute number of pwld in the United Kingdom has been estimated at 2 per cent of the population (Lindsey, 1998). In comparison the number of people suffering from mental illness has been estimated at 4 to 13 per cent of the population. Thus, there are a small number of pwld who require an interpreter. The implication is not that services should not be provided but that the experience of using an interpreter is likely to be minimal for many clinicians. A further issue is that the selection processes are likely to ensure that the people who do finally use a professional service are also experiencing high levels of stress in their relationships. Consequently not only will the clinician have little prior experience, but also interpreting services based typically on the geographical distribution of black and minority ethnic groups will also have little experience of working in services for pwld.

Recent community living options have significantly changed the ways that services are provided. Many pwld within black and minority ethnic families are effectively bilingual with language competence at a similar level for both languages. Fatimilehin and Nadirshaw (1994) conducted a study examining parental attitudes about learning disabilities and found that Asian families reported their sons or daughters speaking both languages with the same level of expressive and receptive oral communication. Thus, a pwld may use English within a service area during the day but at night converse in their family language at home.

Many services for pwld in the UK have been based on the philosophy of normalisation or social role valorisation (e.g. Flynn and Nitsch, 1980; O'Brien, 1981). The interpreter may not understand the effect of the service philosophy when translating questions asked by clinicians. For example, a general assumption is that pwld should be supported with the least restrictive physical and social environment (Landesman-Dwyer, 1985). The concept of the least restrictive environment does not imply a fictitious outcome of 'total independence', but that the least intrusive level of support should be offered, acknowledging that individual need changes over the life course. If the interpreter gave a purely literal translation to a question about living arrangements without regard to the underlying assumptions then the question would potentially be ineffectively expressed. The question could be prejudicial to the needs of the pwld. The significant interaction between the service philosophy and the cultural expectations of the family is subtle and can often be missed.

If the questions posed by the clinician are difficult to translate then the responses by pwld can also be problematic. When choices of substance are being discussed, the assumption that pwld say what they want to say needs to be continually assessed. The presence of social context effects and other cognitive effects require a sensitivity on the part of the interpreter not always required in other interpreting areas. When questions are asked the pwld may experience the tension between 'what I want to say' versus 'what others want me to say' but are without the linguistic skill to indicate that they are experiencing the conflict. The interpreter may then assume that the direct response is the only one that requires interpretation. The effects of social pressure from carers are well documented in the literature. Richardson and Ritchie (1989) in a study of friendships provided many instances of a wide discrepancy between the views of the pwld and their carer(s). For example:

> Susan, aged 33, lived alone with her elderly mother. The mother felt that Susan did not really need friends: 'I don't think it's necessary for her to have a friend. I think I'm her nearest friend and I think that's all she wants.' Yet Susan offered a sharply contrasting view. She had two or three special friends at the Adult Training Centre and, more particularly, a boyfriend. She described with obvious delight the things they did together, the importance of the relationship,

how long she had known him and their intention, supported by an engagement ring, to get married. Her mother knew nothing of the person concerned, of the relationship or of the ring.

(Richardson and Ritchie, 1989: p. 33)

The difference in perspective would not have been highlighted if the interviews had only been conducted at home. Interviews with pwld should be conducted across social environments. Clearly the clinician and interpreter need to confirm the presence (or absence) of social context effects and potentially conduct interviews with others in the social network to evaluate the social context effect. In particular, given that the issues experienced by pwld are not typically with fact finding but in providing explanations for why people act in ways that cause concern, then assessment of the impact of social context is essential.

In addition to social context assessment there are also cognitive effects that require assessment. A major cognitive effect is the 'acquiescence effect' where a pwld is predisposed to say 'yes' even before the question is asked (Sigelman et al, 1981a). In a further study comparing two different question formats Sigelman et al (1981b) concluded that an 'either/or' format was preferable to a 'yes/no' format. Heal and Sigelman (1995) discuss these cognitive effects with recommendations for questioning techniques. The implication of these research findings is that the interpreter may not be aware that the response format chosen by the clinician is a salient factor.

A further consideration is the cognitive bias in perceiving that there are more choices available than there are in actuality. Stancliffe (1995) in a study of 47 pwld still found systematic differences in the perception of choice between themselves and their carers. The results reaffirm the need to undertake questioning across people as well as across environments. The point for the present discussion is to highlight that such a process requires considerably more than one session of interpreter time.

For pwld who have associated mental health problems then the interpreter is also confronted by the variety of expressions that can occur (Borthwick-Duffy, 1994; Sturmey and Sevin, 1993). For example, clinicians are frequently asked to advise carers on how to cope with pwld who are violent towards others. In the questioning it can often lead to the perspective of the pwld being minimised, that is, no account is taken of how the pwld is coping with the situation. A pwld may communicate distress by using non-oral behaviour. The presence of actual physical aggression or self-harm can often distract from assessing both the expressive and the comprehensive dimensions prior to relating recommendations on how to intervene. Hence, the interpreter has to exercise sensitivity in attempting to address both perspectives of the situation.

For people with learning disabilities speech production can also be a factor in the comprehension of speech. The family, irrespective of any cultural considerations, may consider that the content of what the person with learning disabilities is saying is not significant. An assumption that the speech is unintelligible may also be made by, inter alia, the clinician. The use of interpreters, who are not related by family ties, can assist in undertaking a realistic assessment of language competence. Given that the issues for people with learning disabilities are typically not concerned with simple factual information gathering, the use of siblings and other family members as interpreters (similar to other client groups) is not generally recommended.

Given the brief overview of some of the common issues that need to be considered, it appears obvious that a common framework is required to facilitate the interpreting process. In outlining the framework of personal social network analysis, four participants are identified. The pwld; the family/main carers; the interpreter; and the clinician. For linguistic clarity reference will be made to working within a family and not to other living arrangements. However, the ways of working are applicable to other settings. It is also appropriate here to note that the personal social network approach is broadly systemic in orientation. The adoption of a personal social network approach centres the pwld in a set of relationships that form the immediate social environment (Antonucci and Knipscheer, 1990; Wellman, 1988). The immediate social environment typically comprises next of kin and other relationships by marriage. It is unusual for pwld to report many friends in their immediate social network. Pwld, irrespective of cultural and linguistic background, have developmental histories that are qualitatively different from their non-disabled peers. These developmental histories have an enduring and pervasive impact on their personal social networks (Grant, 1993; Krauss et al, 1992).

In the present conceptualisation the role of the interpreter is to negotiate the perceived relations between the various people in the life of the pwld (Kennedy et al, 1990; Laireiter and Baumann,

Table 11.1   Potential shared attributes in the interpreting process

	Pwld	Family	Interpreter	Clinician
Social history	✓	✓	✓	✗
Emotional vocabulary	✓	✓	✓	✗
Cultural stance	✓	✓	✓	✗
Religious affiliation	✓	✓	?	?
Syntax possession	✓	✓	✓	✗
Professional training	✗	✗	✗	✗
Common specific training	✗	✗	✗	✗

Key: ✓ = likely to be shared; ✗ = likely not to be shared; ? = uncertain

1992). The emphasis is on the perceived relations that exist rather than the actual relations that exist (Lakey and Drew, 1997). The present model emphasises the way that pwld construct their personal social network as reported by either speech or diagrams (Raitasuo et al, 1998). It also acknowledges that social network mobilisation as a method can have advantages over the focus on the pwld as having a problem, by giving valued roles to network members and facilitating their participation (e.g. Dunst et al, 1989).

A useful definition for the present purposes is that the interpreter be:

> . . . appropriately interpreting the communications, [and also helping] to bridge cultural value differences between patient and therapist. At times, they set aside the role of interpreter to evaluate the content of what is being translated, and thus fulfill a cultural consultant role.
>
> (Kinzie, 1985)

Table 11.1 outlines some of the key attributes that require attention within the context of the personal social network and the disparity between the various members of the social network. The need for a cultural consultant role is marked.

The application of the framework will be demonstrated using the provision of professional advice in respect of intervention strategies. Cursory inspection of Table 11.1 shows that potentially there are no shared attributes between the clinician and the pwld. Thus, the clinician is likely to feel a sense of powerlessness within the system as a consequence of not sharing these external relations. The feelings generated by the lack of these external relations may also be perceived as deskilling. The salience of these feelings is that if they are not addressed, ideally within supervision, then they are likely to frustrate the contact with the client and lead to premature termination of the involvement. The effect on the family system may be that the clinician overcompensates with respect to the limits of personal knowledge and competence. The family may then attribute 'expert status' to the clinician and marginalise the voice of the pwld. An alternative response might be to consider that a bilingual clinician should be considered. While being an obvious response it nonetheless limits the way that a service may respond and inherently reduces future learning at the individual level.

In the next section each of the key elements identified will be discussed and the implications for practice outlined. It is acknowledged that there are obvious interrelationships between the elements identified. It is acknowledged that the separation is a gross simplification and only exists in order to explain the process.

Social history

The relations between the client and family are likely to be closer to the interpreter by virtue of a shared social history. The personal social network approach makes these shared values a part of the interpreting process. These experiences will potentially include experiences of direct and indirect racism. The form of the questions that are asked should reflect on these issues. Additionally, the distress that is expressed should also be considered within the social context as well as being individualised around the client. The latent value systems within all the participants need to be considered and addressed when framing questions.

The social history will also include elements of familial respect and shame. For example, the asking of insensitive questions, which imply that responsibility for the care of the client can be assigned to social welfare agencies, may lead to future family non-attendance or compliance.

Some families would not perceive similarly direct statements that suggest that the person with learning disabilities is more likely to develop competence outside the family positively. The asking of questions that minimise physical symptoms may also be seen as a failure to understand the issues raised by the family (e.g. Fatimilehin and Nadirshaw, 1994). The perceived failure to offer medication as a remedial measure may result in familial resistance to any intervention. Client gender is also a variable that needs to be understood and addressed within the context of the social history. The social history is not only about past influences (distal) issues, it can also be about recent events. The sensitive questioning about recent major events, for example, weddings, is relevant in gaining a view about how the family are integrated into local social networks. There may be clear care sharing activities that do not need to be replaced but enhanced by additional support, for example, with domiciliary respite care being provided rather than residential care.

Emotional vocabulary

The extent of the shared emotional vocabulary also governs the exchange process. The presence of the interpreter is not only as the bridge for information exchange with a clinician. For example, a care manager might want to share information about how day activities are planned. Using an interpreter to translate the care plan is qualitatively different to sharing an understanding of how emotional issues are being addressed within the family. Knowing how emotional states are ascribed to pwld is crucial in order that statements are made which 'make sense' to the person and the family. The interpreter may challenge some of the statements made by the clinician prior to offering them to the family but the more likely response is to paraphrase and not check back. Critically when direct questions are posed they will relate, in part, to sensitive areas such as personal hygiene, sexual activity and relationships with other service providers. Given that the use of the interpreter is not strictly confined to an information giving and receiving role but that of communicating an analysis of psychological variables, then there is considerable scope for misunderstandings to occur between the clinician and other parties within the system. The client, family or interpreter may not understand the psychological model employed by the clinician. In general, psychological models that problematise the individual and their immediate family are likely to result in lowered uptake of psychological advice and service. There are also other stereotypes, generated and maintained outside services for pwld, that need to be checked personally by the clinician working with black and minority ethnic populations with the interpreter for accuracy and applicability. A preliminary task is to ensure that the emotional vocabulary is explicit. The emotional intelligence of pwld is not generally a direct function of cognitive ability and may be higher than anticipated on the basis of cognitive ability.

Cultural stance

The family are likely to view the use of an interpreter as a linguistic bridge between them and the clinician. The attribution of linguistic skill to the interpreter is also coupled with a tacit assumption that the interpreter is able to undertake the task confidently by virtue of the common language. The question of interpreter confidence is one that needs to be addressed outside the interview situation. An additional attribution sometimes made is that the interpreter can make informed judgments about the significance of the statements made by the client. For example, the question may be asked of the interpreter as to whether the person has learning disabilities. It is not the responsibility of the interpreter to respond to such a question. The interpreter is also in a position relative to his or her own cultural exposure and expectations. These may impose limits on the content of the conversation in ways that do not allow a true reflection of what is being asked and reported back. For example, the client/family may use language misunderstanding as a means of response avoidance. Another salient factor alluded to is the non-oral behaviour that also accompanies the spoken word. For the pwld it may be through being passive that they are able to convey their current psychological state. The issue of confidentiality is also an issue within the cultural stance. The behaviour of the pwld may be spoken of freely within the public context of the family but there may be significant reasons for such information not being available outside the family. The perceived cultural stance of the interpreter may mean that disclosure of familial information is not given. The statements about confidentiality are potentially acknowledged if the clinician makes them. The limits to what is likely to be dis-cussed should also be agreed. There is often an implied assumption that one or two meetings will be sufficient for the work that needs to be undertaken. The formalities may mean that the initial meeting is unlikely to have engaged in more than name sharing and an outline of why the meeting is occurring. A focus on monitoring the pace of the process is also required.

Religious affiliation

On this element there is potentially a difference not only between the clinician but also between the interpreter and the client/family. The extent of a difference should not be overemphasised but nonetheless it can have an effect. For example, there may be conflict between two religious groups that would evidence itself within the context of the dyadic interpreting relationship. The power differential would need to be identified and a resolution negotiated before meaningful discourse could occur. There may be a religious understanding of why the person with learning disabilities has been born and in particular born within the present family. The interpreter, even though they may share the same religion, may not share agreement with the family over specific issues. However, for the clinician a significant action may be not to challenge the view but to be aware of the different explanations that co-exist within the social network. For example, a religious explanation may be that through supporting their disabled offspring atonement for past offences is made by the parents.

Offering domiciliary support for someone who has challenging needs may be perceived as not only inappropriate but also taken as a personal insult since providing personal assistance for their offspring would result in disrespect for their religious belief. However, the offer of different housing arrangements may be more appropriately received. The range and depth of questioning about religious belief is also an area that needs to be considered carefully prior to meeting.

Syntax possession

The existence, possession and use of an alternative syntax may not map easily onto an English syntax. Unless there is adequate pre-preparation the interpretation may be a paraphrase and unclear in its direction. Additionally the pwld may not use the syntax system consistently. As previously discussed, pwld are initially more likely to say 'yes' when asked a direct question of social significance. There is no evidence to suggest that this is not also the case for pwld from black and minority ethnic populations. Therefore the use of syntactical forms, which result in direct questions being asked in translation, should also be avoided. If direct questions are asked then there should be a series of control questions to confirm that the answer is not due to acquiescence. Thus, one key skill in using interpreters is the ability to develop translatable questions. In some instances the exactness of the words used is important. In particular accurate translation of prepositions can be essential for the efficacy of the psychological intervention. The interpreter, unless there has been a pre-meeting, will not necessarily use the most salient word. The use of metaphor also presents difficulties in unprepared translation.

Implications for clinical practice

It is important to restate that the elements presented in Table 11.1 represent one conceptualisation designed to allow examination of the total process. In clinical practice there are necessarily many other factors that operate which cannot be articulated within the confines of the current account. However, it is possible to identify core phases for reflection prior to any significant contact with specific reference to pwld.

The first phase is to determine the position of the clinician within the process of responding to the referral. The use of peer super-vision can facilitate exploration of the therapeutic space that might be available, and allow for consideration of the fact that there may be no equivalent profession in the culture. Furthermore the value of the theoretical processes and their perception can also be discussed. In this phase possible ways of addressing the feelings of being deskilled can be reviewed. Ideally the interpreter shares in the process.

The second phase is to ascertain and obtain information that currently exists from sources who know the family. Typically a significant amount of information is available from generic service provision such as day centres and possibly domiciliary support workers. Within this phase the tendency to label information as culturally specific should be resisted. For example, to consider that the reason a pwld does not attend a day centre may be attributed to an identity problem. The reality may be that there is racist activity within the day centre that the family also shares in a wider social context. Being aware that the distress displayed may be a result of racist experiences is directly relevant to working within learning disability services and is a factor that should routinely be considered. For example, requesting individuals to partake in swimming as a recreational activity may be inappropriate if the session is open to both sexes. The attendant predictable avoidance on those days allocated to swimming cannot be attributed to the individual being phobic or not interested in swimming. Given that the use of information is context dependent, the interpreter can undertake a valuable role in ensuring that the source of the information is clearly ascribed to the social network member. The process is helpful when evaluating possible formulations (Baxter et al, 1990) for the mobilisation of social network support.

The third phase is engagement with an interpreter prior to direct meeting with the pwld. The self-employed nature of the contract held by many interpreters means that there may be difficulties in arranging meetings that are held without the family being present. If there is no in-house provision of interpreting services at least three meetings are essential prior to meeting the referred family. The agenda for these meetings is to examine the power relationships, the intervention process and goals. Attempting to undertake this agenda in 'real time' is likely to result in less effectual working and poorer quality outcomes. A further consideration is that such a practice may engender familial resistance to future meetings if the process is perceived as chaotic and poorly prepared. Within the pre-meetings, mutual exploration of personal perceptions and experience of working with pwld should be scheduled. The opportunity to discuss the technical vocabulary of the clinician should also be planned. Again the content of the processes needs to be addressed before the actual interviews take place. Discussion about the expectations from each meeting is critical to the efficient use of the interpreting service. The timing as to when the meeting should end should also be discussed in advance.

The fourth phase is engagement with the family. The nature of the referral will, in part, direct the actual venue of the family meeting and the relationships that are formed will depend on the preparation that has been undertaken. For example, it may be appropriate in less complex interventions for the interpreter to be seen as offering informational support and for the clinician to be seen as providing access to other sources of support outside the immediate social network.

The therapeutic intervention may be the opportunity for the pwld to have increased social interaction with peers as a consequence of the meeting providing the perceived appropriate support. More complex interventions include the counselling of people with learning disabilities prior to engaging in arranged marriages;

bereavement counselling; counselling sexually abused people; and counselling people with mental health difficulties. While there is evidence that clinical practice encounters these interventions, there is a lack of a literature detailing how these interventions can be understood or facilitated.

The fifth phase is the negotiated withdrawal from the family. A service that relies on interpreters can often result in the abrupt cessation of an intervention. The cessation may be due to a lack of stable funding or to other areas being prioritised by a generically provided service. Families are not necessarily aware of the reasons for cessation but nonetheless are compromised by the outcomes. Pre-planning should account for the length of the involvement of the interpreter and this should be outlined at the beginning of the family meetings. The social network itself may also reject the interpreter because of the identification with the wider social networks that the family participates in. These variables can be discussed prior to direct involvement with the family.

A way ahead

There is a growing acknowledgment within services for pwld that the presence of difference is itself conducive to effecting psychological change. Within the UK there are clearly individuals from black and minority ethnic populations who also are pwld. The importance of ensuring service access for such individuals should be a service priority. However, once accessed the content and meaning(s) of the services provided then become paramount. Clinicians can be part of the process of ensuring that psychological well-being is a consequence of service access. Aspects of the work will require the use of interpreters. At the present time the lack of published literature may not only indicate a low interest but also no conceptual framework of how to ask germane questions. At present, adopting a pragmatic approach when working with a referred family may result in a satisfactory outcome, but is it not time for a more informed perspective so that explanations can be sought when things go wrong?

References

Antonucci, T.C. and Knipscheer, K.C.P.M. (1990) *Social Network Research: Review and Perspectives*. Amsterdam: Swets and Zeitlinger.

Baxter, C., Poonia, K., Ward, L. and Nadirshaw, Z. (1990) *Double Discrimination: Issues and Services for People with Learning Difficulties from Black and Ethnic Minority Communities*. London: Kings Fund Centre.

Borthwick-Duffy, S.A. (1994) 'Epidemiology and prevalence of psychopathology in people with mental retardation'. *Journal of Consulting and Clinical Psychology*, 62: 17–27.

Dunst, C.J., Trivette, C.M., Gordon, N.J. and Pletcher, L. L (1989). 'Building and mobilizing informal family support networks'. In G.H.S. Singer and L.K. Irvin (eds), *Support for Caregiving Families: Enabling Positive Adaptation to Disability*. Baltimore: Paul H. Brookes Publishing.

Fatimilehin, I. and Nadirshaw, Z. (1994) 'A cross-cultural study of parental attitudes and beliefs about learning disability (mental handicap)'. *Mental Handicap Research*, 7: 202–227.

Flynn, R.J. and Nitsch, K.E. (1980) 'Normalization: accomplishments to date and future priorities'. In R.J. Flynn and K.E. Nitsch (eds), *Normalization, Social Integration, and Community Services*. Baltimore: University Park Press.

Grant, G. (1993) 'Support networks and transitions over two years among adults with a mental handicap'. *Mental Handicap Research*, 6: 36–55.

Heal, L.W. and Sigelman, C.K. (1995) 'Response biases in interviews of individuals with limited mental ability'. *Journal of Intellectual Disability Research*, 39: 331–340.

Kennedy, C.H., Horner, R.H. and Newton, J.S. (1990) 'The social networks and activity patterns of adults with severe disabilities: a correlational analysis'. *Journal of the Association for Persons with Severe Handicaps*, 15: 86–90.

Krauss, M.W., Seltzer, M.M. and Goodman, S.J. (1992) 'Social support networks of adults with mental retardation who live at home'. *American Journal on Mental Retardation*, 96: 432–441.

Laireiter, A. and Baumann, U. (1992) 'Network structures and support functions – theoretical and empirical analyses'. In H.O.F. Veiel and U. Baumann (eds), *The Meaning and Measurement of Social Support*. New York: Hemisphere.

Lakey, B. and Drew, J.B. (1997) 'A social-cognitive perspective on social support'. In G.R. Pierce, B. Lakey, I.G. Sarason and B.R. Sarason (eds), *Sourcebook of Theory and Research on Social Support and Personality*. New York: Plenum Press.

Landesman-Dwyer, S. (1985) 'Describing and evaluating residential environments'. In R.H. Bruininks and K.C. Lakin (eds), *Living and Learning in the Least Restrictive Environment*. Baltimore: Paul Brookes Publishing.

Lindsey, M. (1998) *Signposts for Success in Commissioning and Providing Health Services for People with Learning Disabilities*. London: Department of Health.

O'Brien, J. (1981) *The Principle of Normalization: A Foundation for Effective Services.* London: CMH.

Raitasuo, S.J., Taiminen, T. and Salokangas, R.K.R. (1998) 'Social networks experienced by persons with mental disability treated in short-term psychiatric inpatient care'. *British Journal of Developmental Disabilities,* 44: 102–111.

Richardson, A. and Ritchie, J. (1989) *Developing Friendships.* London: Policy Studies Institute.

Sigelman, C.K., Budd, E.C., Spanel, C.L. and Schoenrock, C.J. (1981a) 'When in doubt, say yes: acquiescence in interviews with mentally retarded persons'. *Mental Retardation,* 19: 347–357.

Sigelman, C.K., Budd, E.C., Spanel, C.L. and Schoenrock, C.J. (1981b) 'Asking questions of retarded persons: a comparison of yes–no and either–or formats'. *Applied Research in Mental Retardation,* 2: 347–357.

Stancliffe, R.J. (1995) 'Assessing opportunities for choice-making: a comparison of self- and staff reports'. *American Journal on Mental Retardation,* 99: 418–429.

Sturmey, P. and Sevin, J. (1993) 'Dual diagnosis: an annotated bibliography of recent research'. *Journal of Intellectual Disability Research,* 37: 437–448.

Wellman, B. (1988) 'Structural analysis: from method and metaphor to theory and substance'. In B. Wellman and S.D. Berkowitz (eds), *Social Structures: A Network Approach.* Cambridge: Cambridge University Press.

Chapter 12

Working with the interpreters in adult mental health

Maxwell Magondo Mudarikiri

Introduction

This chapter explores the work of interpreters in adult mental health. The work with interpreters will be thought about from a systemic social constructionist perspective (Cecchin, 1987), and case examples will be used to illustrate some of the points. A systemic perspective is a relational one in that it views people as being active participants within a network of relationships with each other. For instance, significant relationships exist within our families of origin, in our social or community networks, and in our work settings. We all develop patterns of communication that inform and define what any given relationship represents for us. Such patterns of relating and communicating with each other determine the level of intimacy that is permissible within a given relationship. For example, the way we relate to our partner will be very different to how we are with a work superior, which in turn will be very different to how we relate to a total stranger. We are all engaged in a process of evaluating and re-evaluating relationships in our lives. One can therefore imagine the level of complexity involved when an interpreter, a clinician, and a service user are trying to establish a relationship with each other when meeting for the first time. When one views the initial conversation between the clinician, interpreter, and the service user as consisting of a process that involves establishing the parameters of the three-way relationship, then it becomes increasingly important to understand this process from a systemic or relational perspective. In fact the work is as much about understanding the relationships that develop between them as it is about the process of language translation.

From a social constructionist perspective, relationships between people can be thought about as existing within the web of meanings that are created through language. This perspective would argue the case that it is through language that people experience the world, and that it is in this world of language that our relationships, feelings and emotions come to life (Burr, 1995). It is by talking to each other that we socially create, perpetuate and maintain certain meanings or 'truths' about the world and each other. Each different language makes particular meanings possible and allows us to experience certain aspects of ourselves. How we make sense of what we observe is primarily determined by the context in which our observations take place, and the language available to us from which to interpret and give meaning to these observations. Bateson (1972) asserted that context gives meaning to an interaction. Thus one particular description of an interaction between two people in one context may not hold if the same interaction is taking place under very different circumstances. The same may be said for how we attach a particular significance or give meaning to an interaction whilst we are in a conversation with another person (Shotter, 1993); this too will be context dependent. Taking the social constructionist perspective one can view the clinician, the interpreter, and the service user as being involved in an ongoing process of maintaining a relationship with each other within the direct and translated conversations that are possible between them. What they understand of each other will be determined by the context in which their conversation is taking place, as much as how certain expressions and metaphors hold the same meaning when translated across different languages.

Therefore, a systemic social constructionist perspective views people as being actively engaged in relationships with others, which are defined, evaluated, negotiated, re-enacted and lived through the conversations that are possible between them. Language and context have a major bearing on how people make sense of their interactions with and observations of others. For example, seeing a man holding a gun may be understood very differently were this observation to be made in the context of a circus ring, his bedroom, outside a bank, or in the middle of a battle zone. The meaning given to this observation may be very different depending on whether the person observing is a complete stranger to him, his close friend, or his relative. The person observing will only be able to understand this man's actions on the basis of what he or she already knows about him and the nature of any prior relationship between them. If they are total strangers the observer may have to draw on other prior knowledge and life experience in order to make inferences and predict this man's actions. In the process of making the observations and talking with this man, the person observing will inevitably influence what is being observed by virtue of just being there. If this interaction was taking place between a psychiatrist and a suicidal man in the man's home, the interaction between them is likely to be very different to the two of them talking to each other in a circus ring. There is of course always the risk that the suicidal intent of a circus clown may be missed when the gun is being used as part of his regular performance. The same scenario but this time between a police officer and a robber outside a bank may hold very different connotations and may result in a different outcome.

Each person brings his or her understanding of the world and explanatory models for understanding human distress into a relationship. The manner in which the service user's problem is understood will in part be determined by the way in which a shared explanation is developed through the translated conversation (Kaufert, 1990). The interpreter, service user, and clinician will each hold knowledge and understanding that they feel goes some way towards providing an explanation of the service user's difficulties. The bringing forth of an explanatory model that has a good level of consensus between all the parties concerned, will also be determined by the availability of words to describe the service user's psychological difficulties in a particular language. The broader cultural context informs how certain human actions are understood. There is a recursive interplay between language and the cultural context with respect to how each creates particular linguistic expressions and lived experiences of human suffering. The process by which societal consensus is reached about how to understand human actions and suffering is a relational one. Therefore, the systemic constructionist focus is much more on the relational conversations that take place between people. Less emphasis is placed on the representational aspects of language where traditionally greater attention has been placed on the relationship between words and the object that they represent. Riikonen and Smith (1997) say:

Shotter suggests that, *instead of seeking what might be called representational understandings which seek to discover what something is, . . . we may be concerned with the relational understandings which suggest different ways in which we might relate ourselves to our surroundings.*

(Riikonen and Smith, 1997, p. 102)

By privileging a relational understanding of the clinician–interpreter–service user system, it becomes much more possible to think about this work as consisting of co-creating a therapeutic conversation. Each member plays an important part in what becomes available for discussion, and the subsequent understandings that emerge from this conversation.

Systemic social constructionist practice also encourages self-reflexivity on the part of the practitioner (Pearce, 1994). Self-reflexive practice invites the practitioner to develop insight in to how one's own context (e.g. familial, work, social) impacts on the ongoing three-way relationship with the service user and interpreter. Working with an interpreter requires a greater degree of self-reflexivity on the part of the practitioner, as different levels of relationship and communication need to be understood.

Levels of interpretation

The complexities involved with interpretation can be thought about at a number of levels, these being:

1. Linguistic interpretation
2. Metaphorical interpretation
3. Digital interpretation
4. Cultural interpretation

Linguistic interpretation refers to words and their meaning. It is not always possible to find literal translations for words across different languages. The interpreter may have to find alternative words and expressions to convey the meaning behind a particular word or concept that is being used.

Metaphoric interpretation requires the interpreter to draw on his or her contextual knowledge (e.g. culture, class, ethnicity, religion, gender) in order to convey the essence of what is being communicated. Much of everyday and professional language consists of expressions that make use of metaphors. Riikonen and Smith (1997) note the possibility for metaphors to reveal or obscure certain understandings of a concept or phenomenon, when metaphors are transposed and translated from one domain, and examined from the perspective of another domain. The expression 'I have a heavy pain in my heart' may have a literal interpretation that may alert a GP to heart problems if the medical metaphor of symptoms and causes is being drawn on. In some languages this expression may be synonymous with communicating sadness or grief. Within a religious understanding this statement may represent a feeling of guilt and need of atonement.

Digital interpretation refers to non-verbal communication. There are cultural and societal variations in terms of the meanings that are ascribed to certain gestures and non-verbal expressions, as well as what is seen as permissible in particular situations. If the clinician does not ask the interpreter to provide an interpretation of the non-verbal communication, significant communication from the service user may be lost.

Culture can be defined to include practices, beliefs and values that are drawn from historical and contemporary influences associated with race, ethnicity, religion, age, gender, sexuality, and socio-political contexts (Raval, 1996). Pearce (1989) suggests that we learn about culture 'by participating in it and not by studying it'. Pearce goes on to say:

> Culture is precisely this taken for granted aspect of our social worlds that surround relationships, identities, or speech acts that we think about.
>
> (Pearce, 1989, p. 301)

The interpreter therefore plays an important role in helping the service user and the clinician develop a cultural and contextual understanding. An interpreter will often provide an interpretation of what has been said at a cultural level. The interpreter has to make practical and clinical judgements about the timing of when particular levels of interpretation are provided during the course of a session. As many clinicians only emphasise the linguistic level of translation in their work it is not surprising that difficulties arise in the work carried out with interpreters in mental health settings.

Impressions created about working with interpreters

Much of the literature on working with interpreters has highlighted many of the difficulties that arise in this work:

> Sometimes, however, an interpreter only clouds communication and everyone ends up frustrated.
>
> (Grasska and McFarland, 1982, p. 1376)

Grasska and McFarland describe what they call intrinsic and extrinsic problems when the work is being carried out with an interpreter. Intrinsic problems refer to the inherent difficulties that arise in translation and interpretation. Differences in language, culture, ethnicity, and life experience have a bearing on the extent to which a translated conversation is fully understood by the interpreter, clinician, and service user. There will inevitably be aspects of life experience or human distress that are difficult to translate into another language and convey in a way that allows someone else to gain a full understanding of these. One has to simultaneously understand and interpret the literal, non-verbal, cultural and metaphorical meanings that underlie any conversation. We know that even when the same language is shared between people there is no guarantee that they will hold a shared understanding of what has been communicated.

Grasska and McFarland (1982) ascribe the lack of sufficient training for interpreters and clinicians as being associated with the extrinsic problems. The general expectation places the onus on interpreters to be trained, but the same expectation is rarely made of the clinician. It is therefore not surprising that much of the literature tends to focus on the problems that arise in the work with interpreters (Phelan and Parkman, 1995).

Another issue that arises in clinical work is the issue of knowledge and power. Language can play a key role in the process of generating and perpetuating power imbalances, and thereby leading to the inclusion or exclusion of people from particular networks. Pearce (1994) sees power as the 'inclusion or exclusion in and out of conversations'. When working with an interpreter there will be moments in the conversation where the service user, clinician, or interpreter feel included or excluded from the conversation that is taking place between them (Raval, 1996). When people experience a feeling of being excluded there is an increased chance that they will feel unable to challenge this. Alternatively, they may engage in a symmetrical relationship whereby each person becomes more distrusting or undermining of the other. For example, an interpreter may feel unable to caution the clinician about the cultural appropriateness of the mental health interview or diagnosis being made by the clinician about the service user. The interpreter in this situation may then begin to undermine the work of the clinician or form an unhelpful alliance with the service user. Alternatively, an interpreter may be so closely identified with the service user's experience of disempowerment that he or she may not be fully able to get across the service user's point of view to the clinician. There may be occasions when the service user feels excluded, when for example he or she views the interpreter as being in an alliance with the clinician, or instances when the clinician feels excluded when the interpreter and service user are engaged in a long conversation in the service user's first language. The clinician has to work hard to ensure that such negative processes are avoided in the therapeutic work.

The context of interpreting

It is important to take note of the context in which the interpreter's work is being carried out. The task that is set and the role that the interpreter is expected to fulfil are important contextual factors that have to be taken into account. The way an interpreter works when the task is one of making a mental health diagnosis may be very different to when the same interpreter is facilitating ongoing therapy. The interpreter's task is made easier when the clinician ensures that adequate preparation has taken place prior to starting the work. An interpreter needs to be empowered to change the translation if it will convey the intent of the clinician's question more accurately, or to seek clarification from the clinician when this may be required to render the translation meaningful. The interpreter needs time to supplement the clinician's questions in order to elicit useful information from the service user. Phelan and Parkman (1995) say:

> Interpreters should be told to always ask for clarification if something is not clear, rather than guessing what is said.
>
> (Phelan and Parkman, 1995, p. 556)

In the process of therapy it is equally important to minimise ambiguity and both the interpreter and service user need to feel confident in being able to ask the clinician for clarification if this is needed. Ambiguity can arise at a number of different levels. People make sense of communication at an internal level (the conversation that one is having in one's head), an external level (what is being spoken), and at a non-verbal level (e.g. gestures, tone of voice, emotional expression in how something has been said). The interpreter has the unenviable task of rendering a meaningful translation that reflects all the levels at which communication is taking place. The timing of when clarification is sought may also be an important factor that may impede or facilitate the work and the therapeutic relationship. The clinician has to take responsibility from the outset for ensuring that the service user and interpreter feel able to seek out clarification of what is being discussed. The clinician has to ensure that enough time has been allocated in order to carry out the work with an interpreter.

There may also be occasions when being able to remain curious about an ambiguity that has arisen and being able to track this can lead to new helpful insights, rather than trying to insist on a word-for-word translation. Picking up on a misunderstanding may open up new areas for exploration.

The following case example illustrates the importance of the preparation that is necessary when setting up a piece of work with an interpreter.

In meeting with a female service user and a female interpreter, the service user was asked about what she saw as her problems. She seemed to have understood the question asked by me, and immediately began to answer the question using her first language by directing her reply to the interpreter. The interpreter then asked this lady a further question based on her initial reply suggesting that she was experiencing difficulties with her periods and that this was now affecting her marriage. The interpreter was asked by me about the question that she had asked the service user, and the interpreter responded saying that she had asked the service user whether she wished to share this information with me, as she felt that the topic of conversation had been very personal and intimate for the service user.

On reflection this encounter can be thought about through the lens of forming a therapeutic relationship and conversational rules. I had not made time prior to the session to discuss this piece of work with the interpreter and to discuss with her what role she would take on. The interpreter had appropriately protected the service user's interests by seeking out her permission for sharing personal information with me. I had started the session with the assumption that the interpreter would know what she was supposed to do. The interpreter had therefore been required to clarify the boundaries of the therapeutic relationship and the level of intimacy that the service user felt comfortable with given that this was her first appointment with me. Also, I had not determined the level of training or competency of the interpreter prior to starting this piece of work. With hindsight I would have benefited from making adequate time available prior to the start of this session in order to build up a working relationship with the interpreter, and to clarify the roles that each of us would take in the work. I had not created the space to empower the interpreter to make an equal contribution to the work before it was started. The interpreter may not have had a context from which to make sense of the questions that I was asking, and what theoretical ideas were underpinning my questions.

The interpreter as an active participant

There is no active observer to an interaction who does not influence what he or she observes. Therefore, the notion that interpreters can carry out their work as if they have no prior cultural or familial context, or views and opinions is unhelpful. At worst it can be a dangerous view to hold as it generates a model of work where interpreters are seen as having no more than a mechanical translating role in the work. The interpreter will bring their personhood, life experience, and work experience into an encounter with the clinician and service user. Embracing the personal qualities of the interpreter into the work can have an enhancing effect, rather than becoming a problem that has to be overcome. To utilise the interpreter effectively requires training on the part of the clinician.

A model of working is therefore encouraged where the interpreter, clinician and service user feel empowered to play an active and equal role in the therapeutic encounter. This model would view interpreters as bilingual health or social care professionals in their own right.

The clinician, interpreter, and service user may each hold very different understandings or expectations of what the referral to an adult mental health setting will signify and involve. The inclusive model of working encourages interpreters and service users to take on a collaborative, active and more involved role in the work. This may go some way to address the power imbalances. When the work is seen as a three-way process of communication it becomes more possible to explore different understandings of the same observations. It then becomes possible to entertain different explanatory models of the service user's difficulties, and to jointly seek out culturally appropriate solutions to the service user's difficulties. Each of the participants should feel able to make an informed contribution to this work. Allowing for viable alternative viewpoints to emerge through a therapeutic conversation can leave open the way for new understandings to develop in a mutually respectful way (Anderson and Goolishian, 1992). As the ideas that are generated about how best to understand the service user's difficulties are going to be context dependent, the clinician has to be responsible for ensuring that the interpreter and the service user can have a real 'voice' in the work.

Personal and professional narratives

Each one of us draws on certain aspects of our personal and professional narratives, and life experiences when meeting others. A clinician may hold a narrative about his/herself as the professional expert who is expected to make a diagnosis and work out a treatment plan. However, he or she may also be able to draw on personal narratives about him/herself that may bring alternative insights into the work. The interpreter may see his or her role as simply to translate or may feel able to draw on his or her personal and professional experience to work in a broader way. The service user may be drawing on his or her life narrative and cultural beliefs in trying to make sense of his or her psychological distress.

A female service user from the Far East had been admitted onto a psychiatric ward as she was supposedly hearing voices. The clinician had been asked to carry out a diagnostic interview with an interpreter. The interpreter who had considerable experience of working in this service asked the clinician if he could talk with the service user prior to starting the interview in order to gain background information and to set the context of the interview for her. In this con-

versation it emerged that the service user had been feeling low when she had gone to see her GP, and following hospital admission had commented to ward staff with her limited spoken English that the birds were talking to her. On exploring this further the interpreter was told by her about how after migration from a large built up city in her country of origin, the rural hospital setting was so much nicer with the greenery and the trees, and how it had been such a pleasure for her to wake up in the morning and hear the birds singing. In her language this was expressed in a way that she translated into her limited English as 'having the birds talk to her'. The interpreter was able to gain further background history from the service user. On the basis of this information the interpreter suggested to the clinician that the diagnostic interview needed to look at other factors beyond the supposed 'psychotic symptom' of hearing voices (i.e. the birds talking to her).

In many services interpreters are employed as bilingual health workers or health advocates. Within the setting described above the interpreter had the assurance of being able to take on a more independent role, as he had been working with this service for many years. He was able to bring a cultural and linguistic understanding, in addition to his knowledge of adult mental health. This enabled him to get the relevant information from the service user in order to help the clinician with carrying out the diagnostic interview. The preliminary groundwork done by the interpreter had made it easier for the service user to explain her difficulties with more ease to the clinician. The clinician was able to focus on the more relevant aspects of the service user's distress and difficulties. In this instance the interpreter had been able to carry a personal and professional narrative that was supported in the work context. A clinician who may not have worked with this interpreter before could have seen the initial request by the interpreter to talk with the service user alone as undermining or threatening of his or her professional role and identity.

Applying the Milan systemic approach

In the above case example the interpreter was able to use his different position in relation to the work setting and the clinician, to help bring forth a different view and meaning to what had been said by the service user. A discussion with the interpreter prior to starting a session with the service user can be helpful in generating hypotheses and possible explanations for the service user's presenting problems. The author has found the format of the Milan systemic team of organising the time into distinct phases a helpful one (Cecchin, 1987; Palazzoli et al, 1980), along with their ideas of hypothesising, circularity, neutrality and curiosity. The time is organised to allow for a preliminary discussion by the workers to develop provisional ideas about how to understand the service user's difficulties (i.e. the pre-session). This is then followed by the interview with the service user that explores some of the provisional ideas and also allows for new ones as the service user provides further information (i.e. the interview). If there is time the workers may have another discussion after the interview to develop their ideas further before going back to the consulting room with their refined ideas; it is at this point that specific suggestions may be made to the service user about how to manage his or her difficulties. There is further time built in after seeing the service user for the workers to reflect on the session and plan for the next interview with the service user.

In the preliminary discussion with an interpreter it becomes possible to explore potential hypotheses about the service user's difficulties based on the available information given in the referral letter. The interpreter in the role as health advocate and cultural consultant can advise the clinician as to what areas to explore with the service user in a culturally informed, sensitive and appropriate way. The interpreter is able to bring insights from his or her cultural context and life experiences into this discussion. This process also allows the clinician to keep an open mind and retain his or her curiosity, rather than close down the questioning too quickly or become too organised by his or her preconceptions or biases (i.e. trying to maintain a neutral stance and retain curiosity). Taking a relational perspective (i.e. circularity) allows the clinician to think about the service user's difficulties by taking into account how significant other relationships and the context are impacting on the service user's psychological distress. The direction of the work can then be jointly planned between the interpreter and clinician in the initial phase of the work, and hypotheses or areas for further exploration can be developed.

Another viewpoint is obtained when the service user joins the clinician and the interpreter. The service user brings another perspective to the work and needs to be empowered to hold an equitable position in relation to the work. Maintaining a stance of curiosity can help prevent the therapeutic system from becoming too quickly organised into trying to diagnose the problem or find quick solutions before the whole picture has emerged. The therapeutic conversation allows for new meanings and understandings to be developed in this joint endeavour. This also allows for self-reflexivity on the part of all the people making up the therapeutic system.

Following the interview with the service user it is helpful to have a post-session discussion between the clinician and interpreter, in order to clarify information or elaborate on ideas in a way that may not have been possible in direct conversation with the service user. The post-interview discussion also allows for further reflection on the work, and gives the interpreter an opportunity to share observations or insights with the clinician that may not have been possible during the interview, and to plan future work with the service user. A case example is given below to illustrate this approach to working with an interpreter.

Mr B was referred by his GP to a psychiatrist. Mr B had reported experiencing severe anxiety symptoms. Following the psychiatric assessment he was referred to the psychology service for individual counselling. As he had made several references to his marital difficulties during the consultation with the clinician a decision was reached to invite his wife to the next appointment, and as he had said that she did not speak much English an interpreter was invited to the session with the couple. During the session with the couple it was noticeable that Mr B showed a preference to talk to his wife through the interpreter when he was invited to explain his feelings directly to her. His wife answered the questions using both her first language and English. She was quite tearful and upset by her husband's difficulties, but described the difficulties as being caused by the stress on her husband, related to the tensions between them as a result of his parents spending too much time with them. His parents lived next door to them and the family ate their meals together, leaving little time that the couple could be alone. She felt that she was mostly confined to the kitchen as her father-in-law liked to sit in the living room, and out of respect she was expected not to be in the presence of her father-in-law. Mr B felt that as his parents were old and because his mother had poor sight he should be there to look after them. He was beginning to question his potency in being able to provide for his whole family. Mrs B began to direct her conversation more and more to the interpreter as this particular session progressed.

During the post-session discussion with the interpreter it was possible to unravel the different possible understandings about this couple's situation, and the dynamics that had been taking place in the consulting room. The alliance that Mrs B had formed with the interpreter was discussed, and the positives and negatives of this relationship were thought about. The interpreter's cultural insights proved useful in understanding the difficulties being experienced by Mrs B. The interpreter pointed out the class and caste differences between the couple and how she was closer in her own background to Mrs B. Thought was also given to how the interpreter could hold a position of curiosity and not become too closely allied with Mrs B. The clinician was able to discuss the dynamic process where the interpreter may have been put in the position of 'rescuer' by Mrs B, and possibly lose her connection with Mr B. Developing a relational hypothesis helped with getting a better understanding of how the family context was influencing the couple's relationship, and how this was impacting on his anxiety symptoms. The interpreter had also been sensitive to the issues for Mr B, and was able to develop a hypothesis about how his role in the family may have been eroded due to him having to take early retirement from his work in his early 40s as a result of his anxiety symptoms, which had started when he was given a promotion that he had not wanted. Having the interpreter as an ally in the early stages of the work enabled Mrs B to talk more directly in English with the clinician in subsequent sessions, and it seemed that having the interpreter present for every session had helped her find a 'voice' in this work. The interpreter was older than Mr and Mrs B and her age may have been a helpful factor in this work. She had experienced similar familial dilemmas to those being experienced by the couple, and the couple may have been able to draw on her life experience and wisdom in helping them resolve their dilemmas. The interpreter may have straddled the 'traditional and modern' positions in a way that was helpful for this couple. Having the interpreter present had enabled the couple to converse in a way that may have not been possible had the couple been seen without the interpreter.

Summary

This chapter has drawn on a systemic social constructionist approach in developing the clinical work carried out with the help of an interpreter. The approach utilises the structure of carrying out clinical work that has been developed by the Milan group of systemic therapists, and the author has found the time built in for a pre-session and post-session discussion with the interpreter to be invaluable in his work. The presence of the interpreter is seen as an active one in which he or she is able to bring another perspective to that held by the clinician and service user. With the help of the interpreter it is possible to develop levels of understanding that go beyond the literal translation, and thereby co-construct therapeutic conversations which allow reflexive space for meanings and new insights to evolve in the process of therapy.

References

Anderson, H. and Goolishian, H. (1992) 'Client is the expert'. In S. McNamee and K. Gergen (eds), *Therapy as a Social Construction*. London: Sage.

Bateson, G. (1972) *Towards an Ecology of Mind*. St Albans: Chandler Publishing Company.

Burr, V. (1995) *An Introduction to Social Constructionism*. London: Routledge.

Cecchin, G. (1987) 'Hypothesizing–circularity–neutrality revisited: an invitation to curiosity'. *Family Process*, 26: 405–413.

Grasska, M.A. and McFarland, T. (1982) 'Overcoming the language barrier: problems and solutions'. *American Journal of Nursing*, September, 82(9): 1376–1378.

Kaufert, J. (1990) 'Sociological and anthropological perspectives on the impact of interpreters on clinician/client communication'. *Sante Culture Health*, VII (2–3): 209–235.

Palazzoli, S., Boscollo, L., Cecchin, G. and Prata, G. (1980) 'Hypothesizing–circularity–neutrality: three guidelines for the conductor of the session'. *Family Process*, 19: 3–12.

Pearce, W.B. (1989) *Communication and the Human Condition*. Southern Illinois: University Press.

Pearce, W.B. (1994) *Interpersonal Communication: Making Social Worlds*. London: Harper Collins.

Phelan, M. and Parkman, S. (1995) 'How to do it. Work with an interpreter'. *British Medical Journal*, 311: 555–557.

Raval, H. (1996) 'A systemic perspective on working with interpreters'. *Clinical Child Psychology and Psychiatry*, 1: 29–43.

Riikonen, E. and Smith, G.M. (1997) *Re-Imagining Therapy – Living Conversations and Relational Knowing*. London: Sage.

Shotter, J. (1993) *Conversational Realities*. London: Sage.

Chapter 13

The refugee context and the role of interpreters

Rachel Tribe and Jean Morrissey

Introduction

The processes of migration to the UK can present many different experiences and dilemmas. Some of the dilemmas frequently experienced by refugees differ significantly from other migrant groups and may have adverse effects on refugees' mental well-being. Traditions of help-seeking behaviour for emotional or family dilemmas among some refugee groups may display themselves in many different ways. These different traditions might be viewed as more important when a common spoken language is not shared and communication is through an interpreter. Within the domain of mental health, interpreters offer a valuable and skilful service and can play an important role in bridging the gap between client and health practitioner.

This chapter will explain some of the differences between refugees and other migrant groups. An overview of refugee migration processes to the UK will be provided, followed by a general overview of some of the dilemmas frequently experienced by refugees. Different models of help-seeking behaviour in dealing with emotional problems will be discussed. Differences which a refugee may experience in accessing mental health services via an interpreter will be considered, as well as the specific issues an interpreter and mental health professional will need to consider when working with refugees.

Overview of refugee migration patterns to the UK

Refugees differ significantly from other immigrant groups in that other groups have usually made a positive choice to migrate and change their country of residence. As a result, they have generally been able to plan the move systematically over time. In contrast, refugees usually have to flee at short notice for fear of their lives and often to unknown destinations.

A refugee in Britain is someone who has obtained refuge under the terms of the 1951 United Nations Convention Relating to the Status of Refugees which defines refugees as:

> People who, because of a well-founded fear of persecution, for reasons of race, religion, nationality, membership of a particular social group or political opinion, leave their country of origin and are unable or unwilling to avail themselves of the protection of that country.

An asylum-seeker is someone who has applied for refugee status and is waiting for a decision to be made by the Home Office. Many asylum-seekers will have gone through immensely traumatic experiences prior to leaving their country of origin; this is why they are applying for asylum in Britain. Interpreters may be used at a variety of points in the process. These may range from the initial interview at the airport or other point of entry, to a variety of different stages in the asylum legal procedure and beyond.

Refugees come to Britain from over forty-one countries (Home Office, 1999). In 2001, people claiming asylum in Britain numbered 71,700 (Home Office, 1999). Within this group, every continent was represented and at least fifty different languages were spoken by asylum-seekers on entering Britain.

An individual who has received full refugee status under the UN Convention, as determined by the United Kingdom (UK) Immigration and Nationality Department, is entitled to live in the UK as long as they wish. A status giving fewer rights is named 'Exceptional Leave to Remain' (ELR). This means that the individual has been granted permission to remain in the UK on humanitarian grounds. The Home Office reasoning behind this status is that it is currently inappropriate for the asylum-seeker to return to their country of origin, however if the situation changes the asylum-seeker will be expected to return, although after 7 years (4 in the pending legislation), he or she can apply for indefinite leave to remain.

The period between applying for asylum and receiving an initial decision varies between being the same day, in very exceptional cases, to 3–4 years, with the average period being 12 months

(Refugee Council, 1998). Many people will not be successful or will be involved in lengthy appeal procedures and some eventually will be returned to their country of origin. The 1999 Immigration and Asylum Act is to be superceded by the Nationality, Immigration and Asylum Bill, 2002 which is currently before Parliament. The government claims that this legislation will speed up the process to under 6 months. The period awaiting a decision, or undergoing the appeal procedures may be an extremely gruelling and uncertain time for an asylum-seeker. These difficulties may be exacerbated for an asylum-seeker whose language is not English, as they will be further distanced from the procedure by having to use an interpreter as their *voice* throughout this difficult period.

Locating in the UK

All refugees and asylum-seekers are likely to face a range of dilemmas and difficulties in the UK, which in turn may add to the traumas already experienced. On becoming an asylum-seeker, an individual is likely to be faced with a number of losses. These may include loss of a common language and therefore the ability to communicate and be understood by those around them. This can be a frightening and disempowering experience. Other major losses may include contact with loved ones, home, job, and culture (Richman, 1998; Tribe and Shackman, 1989). An additional loss may be the view of their anticipated future and life plans.

The following account is an example of the psychological effects of becoming a refugee for one client seen in an agency specialising in providing services to asylum-seekers. Mr Ali, a refugee from Iraq, gave the following self-description of feeling 'infantalised' by the experience of becoming a refugee. His account was given with the help of an interpreter.

I used to be a strong and potent man who could look after myself and my family. Here I feel like a naughty and frightened child. I have no idea what tomorrow or my future may bring. I fear I could be deported at any time, I am unsure if the British will let me stay, as I told my story to a friend and he translated it into English and wrote it on to the asylum form. I don't know him very well, I met him on the bus as I could tell he was from my country. I can't tell if he can speak English properly himself and if he wrote everything I told him down. I also don't know if he is a political man and may report me to my government and cause trouble for my family. I feel everywhere I go I have to beg for everything.

The largest proportion of asylum-seekers (80 per cent) are single people (Refugee Council, 2001) and unaccompanied children are an important group. Asylum-seekers may have no support network, family members or access to people who speak the same language. They are therefore unable to talk to people who can help them make sense of their new situation in Britain, including the legal process and the very different cultural context. Many refugees would like nothing more than to return to their country of origin if it were safe for them to do so. Thus it might be argued that refugees are likely to be highly vulnerable to emotional distress, given their previous traumatic experiences in their countries of origin, and the uncertainty and unsettling nature of becoming a refugee in a different country and continent (Kelly, 1994; Carey-Wood et al, 1995; Williams, 1989).

Lavik et al (1997) found a complicated relationship among refugees in Norway between demographic background, traumatisation, exile situation, symptoms and social functioning. Not speaking the dominant language of the country in which one is currently based means that even conducting day-to-day matters becomes extremely difficult and complicated. These difficulties may be further exacerbated by difficulties in accessing mental health services and interpreters when resettled (Gong-Guy et al, 1991).

Social support as a protective variable

Social support has been shown to be a protective factor in emotional well-being (Brown and Harris, 1978; Gorst-Unsworth and Goldenberg, 1998). This has implications for the newly arrived asylum-seeker and their mental health. It has also been suggested that social support may offer some kind of long-term protection to psychological health (Davidson, 1980; Ressler et al, 1988). Allodi (1989) noted that social support from the cultural community and receiving society may enhance adaptation. Indeed Bisson and Deahl (1994) go so far as to suggest that social support in the presence or absence of other factors may be more important in the presence (or otherwise) of traumatic reactions than the provision of psychological interventions soon after the event. McCallin and Fozzard (1990) claimed that perception of family members as sources of support significantly predicted psychological adjustment among Mozambican refugees. Additionally, Hobfoll et al (1991) claim that supporting others may benefit not only the recipient but also the giver.

If asylum-seekers are separated from their family and community this in itself may have detrimental effects on their emotional well-being (Tribe, 1999a,b; Woodcock, 1995). Lopez et al (1988), working with an established Chilean refugee community in the USA, found that one of the two most pertinent factors mentioned was the lack of a mutual support system, while loneliness was mentioned as a recurring difficulty by the research participants. The importance of linking with others for social support has also been stressed by Light (1992), Tribe and Shackman (1989), and Venables and Rodriquez (1989).

Recent changes in the legislation and the concomitant negative publicity may have led to antipathy towards asylum-seekers and refugees from members of the receiving society. Asylum-seekers and refugees may also be subject to racism and have no right to work or claim welfare benefits. The 1999 Immigration and Asylum Act is to be superceded by the Nationality, Immigration and Asylum Bill, 2002. This is currently before Parliament. The European Monitoring Centre on Racism and Xenophobia, which is based in Vienna, undertook research into attitudes towards asylum-seekers. They criticised the British media for their 'xenophobic and intolerant coverage of asylum issues' (Racism and Cultural Diversity, 2002).

Refugees and mental health categorisation

There appears to be a body of literature claiming to show a correlation between becoming a refugee and psychological health difficulties. Given the considerable losses and associated changes which many refugees experience this is perhaps inevitable (Eisenbruch, 1991; Tribe, 1999b; Van der Veer, 1992). Early studies of refugees and mental health were conducted in the post-World War II period, when movement of refugees on a significant scale took place. Studies conducted by Eitinger (1959) in Norway, Krupinski and Stoller (1965) in Australia, and Murphy (1955) in Britain, all suggested a link between psychiatric disorder and refugee status. The three studies found significantly higher rates of psychiatric disorder compared to the native populations, for periods of up to 10 years after migration.

Several explanations for differences in the prevalence of mental illness among refugees have been suggested. Furnham and Bochner (1986) and Oberg (1960) have written about the idea of cultural shock as a stress response to a new and different culture. However, Coelho and Ahmed (1980) have claimed that this is frequently associated with reactive mental disorders. For many refugees, internal representations of the world with respect to which identity has been developed, are almost consistently challenged by the instability and changes in their external world. This may leave little stable ground for (re)constructing either a coherent self-image or for attempting goal-directed behaviour (Ager, 1994). Gorst-Unsworth and Goldenberg (1998) have written about the importance of meaning and existential factors associated with exile for each refugee and their subsequent role as mediating variables.

Eisenbruch (1991), working with Cambodian refugees, developed the term 'cultural bereavement', which is defined as encompassing the loss of previously held social networks, self-identity and cultural values. He claims that this may lead refugees to 'live in the past'. He is concerned that mental health practitioners trained in western mental health diagnosis may be too keen to diagnose, when the symptoms may be a way of dealing with the issues.

> If western mental health professionals try to identify and treat refugees according to criteria such as those listed in the Diagnostic and Statistical Manual, they run the risk of treating an illness which the refugee does not have, and may leave him or her feeling confused. Such misunderstanding of refugees' needs could be avoided if more emphasis were placed on the cultural meanings of the information gathered from the refugees themselves, even if these may at first seem bizarre to the professional.
>
> (Eisenbruch, 1991, p. 25)

There are a range of arguments about the appropriateness of the diagnostic category Post-Traumatic Stress Disorder (PTSD) in this context. A full discussion of this issue is unfortunately outside the scope of this paper, but interested readers are referred to Bracken and Petty (1998) and de Silva's chapter in Yule (1999) for further discussion of these issues.

Moreover, recent studies that have been mainly focused on Post Traumatic Stress Disorder (PTSD) have attested to increased risk of mental health problems among refugees. For example, Mollica et al (1987) claimed that 92 per cent of refugee patients attending their psychiatric clinic in the USA met diagnostic criteria for PTSD. However, Kinzie and Sack (1991), working interestingly and unusually with a non-clinical refugee sample, found 50 per cent of their high school sample met the PTSD criteria. Clearly, there is no simple explanation for these differential rates.

Zur (1996) writes of some of the difficulties and appropriateness of exporting the western concept of Post Traumatic Stress Disorder (PTSD) to non-western cultures, as do Bracken (1998) and Summerfield (1998). It has been argued that refugees are not in a post-traumatic situation when they start to settle in the west, but in a continuing traumatic situation (Richman, 1998). Moreover, Lewis-Fernandez and Kleinman (1995) challenge the failure of cultural validation of the Diagnostic Statistical Manual (DSM-IV) (American Psychiatric Association, 1994) and the lack of concern around this and related issues. Fuller (1993) found that many of the mental health staff working in Denmark lacked in-depth familiarity of PTSD, its relevance to refugee trauma, methods for working with trauma survivors, countertransference issues, refugee acculturation patterns and cross-cultural psychology. It might be inferred that a similar pattern could be found in other refugee-receiving countries. Racism and issues of difference, and lack of understanding about cultural variables are likely to be important variables in the above findings. These issues have been discussed by a number of writers, including Fernando (1995) and MacLachlan (1997). Given the significance of the above issues, without access to interpreters, many refugees will have no recourse to mental health services, or opportunity for their explanatory health beliefs to be understood.

Interpreters play a vital role in ensuring that non-English speaking asylum-seekers are not barred from accessing health services, including mental health and social service provision. Interpreters may also play a major role in helping asylum-seekers and refugees link up to relevant local networks and to a range of other state provisions, including primary health care services. Many of the specific issues relating to best practice in working with interpreters have been documented in Chapter 7 of this book by Granger and Baker, and will not be re-iterated here. Suffice to say that interpreters may play an indispensable role in mental health assessments and in ensuring that access to mental health services is possible.

Different traditions of help-seeking behaviour and sources of help in dealing with mental health issues

The organising concepts and explanatory health beliefs for a refugee may bear little resemblance to those held by mental health practitioners trained and conditioned into a set of western explanatory health beliefs. Additionally, mental health practitioners may assume that the latter beliefs are generalisable, whereas in reality they are culture-bound (Bracken, 1998; Kleinman, 1980; MacLachlan, 1997; Sue et al, 1988; Zur, 1996).

The idea of having mental health or emotional problems is seen as stigmatising in most of the world. The role of a mental health professional may not be culturally synonymous for many refugees. A senior family member, traditional healer, community elder, allopathic doctor or other person may have held this position; whereas in Britain, there may be few people who can fit this role. For many refugees, they may not even be aware that help with psychological or family difficulties is available as it may be 'packaged' so differently. Moreover, such sources of help may be further distanced from a refugee client who is accessing the service via an interpreter.

The following brief case history illustrates how one client believed that having emotional dilemmas was viewed as unacceptable by his peers.

Pedro, a refugee from Latin America, once came flying into my office several minutes after our session had finished in a highly anxious and aroused state. He told me he had bumped into a friend Enriques in the corridor. He begged me to tell Enriques that his appointment with me was in connection with an arm injury and to say nothing of any emotional dilemmas. It appeared that it was fine to have physical health problems, but to have psychological ones was not acceptable as it was viewed as a stigma.

A number of centres in refugee-receiving countries have attempted to set up a range of psychological and on occasions psycho-social, medical or social welfare services that are culturally appropriate. It is pertinent to ask if anything can be learned from this experience. Boehnlein et al (1985b) and Mollica et al (1987) claim that settings that contain both 'medical and psychotherapeutic or support services' have reported positive results, as measured by attendance and outcome. However, it is not uncommon for clients to still possess considerable anxieties relating to their physical health (Hough, 1991; Tribe, 1998). Hough (1991) claims that refugees' most frequently recorded presenting problems are somatic.

Given the western ideas encapsulated in the idea of therapy and much of mental health provision, for some refugee clients it may seem extremely strange to be asked to talk about thoughts and feelings to a total stranger. Moreover, it may be even more daunting when done through an interpreter. This is one possible reason why the combination of medical and support services plus psychotherapeutic services has been found to be more effective. It is often much safer to exhibit a physical symptom, than talk about the immense pain, anguish and fears that can be felt.

Landy (1977) notes that within a place where health pluralism (a variety of health models) is present, the cultural and social aspects of treatment are equally important. The explanatory model held by the patient may well determine where they seek help for emotional or physical distress (Helman, 1984). Different explanatory health beliefs are likely to contain beliefs about aetiology, epidemiology and cure.

Any type of mental health intervention may be shunned as it may be seen as stigmatising to all the family members. Ideas and beliefs relating to heredity or causality may be different and may not marry well with western ideas of therapy, and individual notions of choice, personal development and causality. Chung and Lin (1994) carried out an interesting study which examined the help-seeking behaviour of 2,777 South East Asian refugees in their native country and how this compared with their behaviour in America. They found that there was a significant difference between use of traditional medicine in their home country and a higher use of western medicine in the USA. Moreover, traditional medicine continued to be important for all the five South East Asian refugee groups after resettlement.

Fernando (1995), Lago and Thompson (1996), Lau (1985) and Tribe (1999a) have all written about the relationship between psychological therapy and culture, noting that the relationship between a culture and its healing rituals is a complex one. The methods which people use to maintain their psychological equilibrium and to find help are in large part developed and defined by the cultural, societal and health rules and meanings these are ascribed in their 'world'. Other authors have also noted that how different cultures will define different behaviours/feelings can be problematic, both for the client and mental health practitioner (Torrey, 1972; Herr, 1987; Westwood, 1990). Interpreters play an important role in bridging the gap between client and clinicians particularly when different traditions of help-seeking behaviour for emotional/family dilemmas may be present.

The language of psychology and mental health

The language of psychology and mental health has been largely based on a western vocabulary and, as the post-modernists have pointed out, language is not a transparent medium as was previously assumed. Words relating to psychiatric, trauma, psychological, counselling/therapy, stress and mental health may not exist or have the same meaning or resonance in other languages. Although the developing multicultural movement accepts that multiple belief systems and perspectives are possible (Highlen, 1997; Sue et al, 1988), language is an ever changing medium that may reflect the dominant cultural beliefs held at any time. Different language codes and usage will always be found between different groupings, as it is a living and ever changing medium. The French spoken in France and that spoken in the République démocratique du Congo (an ex-Belgian colony formerly named Zaire) may be very different, the latter having been enriched by words from one of the four native or indigenous languages. Thus, an interpreter from France and a client from the Congo may speak different variations of the same language. This needs to be considered when looking for an interpreter for a client from the Congo. Although French is the official language of the Congo, many people do not speak it at home; therefore if a refugee has not been fortunate enough to receive much formal schooling they may not be fluent in French. If an immigration interview is undertaken when a French interpreter is used for a Congolese client they may be unable to explain much of their history and might therefore be refused asylum in Britain.

The value and role of interpreters

The benefits of using interpreters for non-English speaking clients has been well documented by Hillier et al (1994), Kline and Spevak

(1980), and Raval (1996), among others. The literature also documents potential dilemmas in working with this non-traditional triad. These problems need to be considered before undertaking mental health work using interpreters if the potential outcomes of the work are to be maximised (Freed, 1988; Harvey, 1984; Owan, 1985; and Tribe, 1998). If these issues are dealt with adequately there is no doubt that an interpreter can provide an essential link between the mental health practitioner and the client seeking consultation and help.

The NHS and other services within Britain employ 'link workers or health advocates' to help health teams try and deliver health provision in a culturally appropriate manner. When working well this is an extremely helpful model. Unfortunately it has not always worked as well as it might, with link-workers often finding that their position and role is either ascribed low status by other health workers or found to be ambiguous. Link-workers are employed to act as patients' verbal advocates in their dealings with health workers. Many link-workers have frequently reported that they are not ascribed a clear role by other health professionals and are used merely as interpreters (Tribe and Sanders, 2003). For a fuller discussion of this issue see Tribe and Sanders (2003).

Interpreters and mental health

As detailed earlier when working with refugees, a shared language and set of cultural understandings may not exist. Interpreters need to play a prominent and important role in ensuring that access to services is not limited by language fluency. Ultimately the best answer may be for a fellow national mental health practitioner to work alongside the refugee client. Unfortunately in many refugee-receiving countries and refugee camps this is not available yet.

Shackman (1984) writes of the dearth of trained mental health interpreters in Britain, with many people having to rely on untrained volunteers or someone in their family/community network. There are many difficulties associated with this situation. Using interpreters in mental health work is never easy, and needs particular sensitivity and ideally training of both parties if it is to work (Tribe and Sanders, 2003). Marcos (1979) writing in New York, stated that all the psychiatrists who participated in his study regarded working with interpreters as difficult, and reported a number of dilemmas. The task of the interpreter is a complex and sophisticated one requiring a range of skills beyond just the ability to speak two languages fluently. He claimed that the following conditions of the interpreter would further distort the process:

- Lack of language competence and language skills
- Lack of psychiatric knowledge
- Attitudes (for example over identification with the client).

Sabin (1975) argues that the patient's emotional suffering and despair may be selectively underestimated in the process of interpretation. While words and meanings are often not interchangeable between languages, interpreters may have to mediate between the two. Hoffman writing in *Lost in Translation* notes:

> River in my language was a vital sound, energised with the essence of riverhood, of my rivers, of being immersed in rivers. 'Rivers' in English is cold – a word without an aura, it has no accumulated associations for me, and it does not give off the radiating heat of connotation.
>
> (Hoffman, 1989, p. 47)

The difficult process of collecting histories through an interpreter has been cited by Hitch and Rack (1980) as leading to the recognition of psychotic and paranoid symptoms and the common misdiagnosis of the client as being schizophrenic. McIvor (1994) has discussed the role of the interpreter in dealing with patients suffering from traumatic stress reactions and other psychological difficulties in a bicultural setting and the associated dilemmas which may arise. Trauer's (1995) study of the utilisation of public psychiatric services in an area of Australia found that although the use made of interpreters was variable, generally there was low use made of interpreters. This study also found that non-English speaking patients had longer median stays in psychiatric hospitals, and that their consultation time was 5 to 10 minutes less than English speakers. Non-English speaking patients were also less likely to be hospitalised voluntarily.

Working with interpreters

The use of interpreters or bicultural workers may change the idiom of work (Tribe, 1998). The pitfalls of working with interpreters/

bicultural workers are many and require training and skill acquisitions by both the therapist and the interpreter. This has particular relevance for displaced people or refugees who may be traumatised and unfamiliar with the British health care setting and explanatory health beliefs. It is important to realise that working with interpreters and people holding different health beliefs can be an extremely enriching and positive experience. Mental health practitioners may need to question their assumptions and traditional ways of thinking.

Raval's (1996) study noted that some mental health workers reported that using an interpreter enabled them to be more reflective in their practice. This in turn enhanced their work in that clients felt freer in talking about their cultural and religious beliefs. However, the majority also reported that an exception to this was when the mental health practitioner was looking for psychotic symptoms or for child sexual abuse. Kline, Acosta and Williams (1980) noted that patients interviewed with interpreters felt understood and wished to return, while the mental health professionals who worked with interpreters in this study hypothesised that these patients would feel less understood and would not wish to return.

The difficulties surrounding issues of trust for refugee clients

Self-disclosure and openness in communication take on a totally different resonance for these clients compared to other client populations. Indeed, such characteristics may have led them to being imprisoned in the first place. Clients may not trust the bicultural worker because they may assume that their compatriot has different political views to their own. For someone coming from a repressive regime, information is an extremely dangerous thing and could place family members remaining in the country of origin at risk of torture, imprisonment or both.

Issues which may require consideration when working with refugees (Tribe, 1998) include the following:

- The client may be separated from their community or reference group and the interpreter may help bridge the gap in some way.
- Having a fellow national or member of a familiar community (as an interpreter/bicultural worker or mental health

professional) may increase the feelings of trust and belonging which the client may feel with the agency, worker and perhaps beliefs about their efficacy.

- It has been suggested by Saxthorp and Christiansen (1991), writing about Middle Eastern refugee families living in exile in Denmark, that interpreters may act as a positive role model for clients.

If working therapeutically using an interpreter with a client the following factors may also need to be considered:

- Issues of transference when a third member is brought into the consultation.
- The interpreter/bicultural worker can inadvertently become part of the therapeutic system.

Other important issues to consider when working with refugees using interpreters

Which model of interpreting (linguistic, advocacy or professional team member model) is used by the agency will always be a variant in the process. Interpreters often feel they are in some way acting on behalf of one or other of the parties (client or practitioner), rarely for both. The way this is initially negotiated is extremely important in ensuring that the session runs smoothly and the three parties are clear about their roles and boundaries. The client may believe that as they share a language, culture and maybe politics with the interpreter, they will automatically be their advocate whereas the interpreter may believe that the contract is merely to interpret the language and may not wish to do any more than this. Given the particular circumstances of refugees these issues may be particularly pertinent. When working with refugees interpreters may find themselves put under pressure to be an advocate as well as an interpreter. Alternatively, the interpreter may believe that they are representatives of the organisation or mental health agency and therefore share a primary alliance with the worker. Clearly, when the traditional consultation moves from a dyad to a triad the dynamics inevitably change.

The cultural understanding which the bicultural worker brings into the therapeutic communication may bridge the gap between health professional and client. It may also enhance the health professional's understanding of the client's history and culture and enable a piece of health provision to be accessed by the client, which might not have been possible without the interpreter's work (Raval, 1996; Tribe, 2002).

In the west or in the major refugee-receiving countries, some centres for asylum-seekers and refugees are fairly well established. They also bear a number of different relationships to the authorities, who hold responsibility for the giving of asylum, or full refugee status. Nafsiyat (an intercultural centre in London) is doing exceptional work in providing psychotherapy services to ethnic groups including refugees, as are a number of other organisations. However, it might be argued that services for less visible or less dramatically traumatised refugees have been less successful in becoming established unless they are working with one particular refugee group. This may be due to reasons of securing funding. It may also reflect the ambivalence felt by much of the population concerning asylum-seekers/refugees or the importance of psychological help. When these two components are coupled together, plus the potential ambivalence of refugees to use them given their unknown status to the 'authorities', it may be extremely difficult for such resources to become established. Moreover, these difficulties may be further exacerbated when different languages are spoken and access is therefore difficult.

There is an enormous amount of quite exceptional work that often goes unannounced, as is the work done by refugee community groups, often with very little in the way of resources. The number of clients helped by these groups is probably larger than those assisted by 'official agencies'. The commitment, motivation and skills exhibited by those who work with large numbers of refugees in these groups should not be ignored. These groups may on occasions appear more approachable, as the newly arrived refugee knows that her/his language will be spoken, and cultural mores understood. Additionally, the client will probably not have the same concerns that the organisation could be linked to the government and therefore to the giving or withholding of resources.

Summary

In summary, this chapter has examined the legal definitions for the award of refugee status in Britain. Brief data on refugees to Britain was presented together with some of the legalities concerning this process. The need for trained interpreters at a number of points in this process was identified. Research on refugees and mental health was examined, as was the need to recognise different explanatory health beliefs among different refugee groups. Particular attention was drawn to the number of complex issues that may arise when working with an interpreter for refugee clients. Clearly, working with a non-traditional triad presents many challenges for all participants in the consulting room. Failure to address such issues may impede both access to help and the potential for a successful outcome with this client group.

References

Ager, A. (1994) 'Mental health issues in refugee populations: a review'. Working Paper of the Harvard Center for the study of Culture and Medicine, Harvard Medical School, Dept of Social Medicine.

Allodi, F. (1989) 'The psychiatric effects in children and families of victims of political persecution and torture'. *Danish Medical Bulletin*, 27: 229–232.

American Psychiatric Association (1994) *Diagnostic and Statistical Manual of Mental Disorders* (4th edn). Washington DC: American Psychiatric Association.

Bisson, J. and Deahl, M.P. (1994) 'Psychological debriefing and prevention of post-traumatic stress – more research is needed'. *British Journal of Psychiatry*, 165: 717–720.

Boehnlein, J.K., Kinzie, J.D., Ben, R. and Fleck, J. (1985) 'One-year follow-up study of posttraumatic stress disorder among survivors of Cambodian concentration-camps'. *American Journal of Psychiatry*, 142 (8): 956–959.

Bracken, P. (1998) 'Hidden agendas: deconstructing post traumatic stress disorder'. In P. Bracken and C. Petty (eds) *Rethinking the Trauma of War* (pp. 38–60). London: Free Association Books.

Bracken, P. and Petty, C. (1998) (eds) *Rethinking the Trauma of War*. London: Free Association Books.

Brown, G. and Harris, T. (1978) *The Social Origins of Depression*. London: Tavistock Publications.

Carey-Wood, J., Duke, K., Karn, V. and Marshall, T. (1995) *The Settlement of Refugees in Britain*. London: HMSO.

Chung, R.C.Y. and Lin, K.H. (1994) 'Help-seeking behaviour among South East Asian refugees'. *Journal of Community Psychology*, April, 22 (2): 109–120.

Coelho, G.V. and Ahmed, P. (1980) (eds) *Uprooting and Development*. New York: Plenum Press.

Davidson, S. (1980) 'The clinical effects of massive psychic trauma in families of holocaust survivors'. *Journal of Marital and Family Therapy*, 6(1): 11–24.

De Silva, P. (1999) 'Cultural aspects of post-traumatic stress disorder'. In W. Yule (ed.), *Post-Traumatic Stress Disorders, Concepts and Therapy*. Chichester: John Wiley.

Eisenbruch, M. (1991) 'From post traumatic stress disorder to cultural bereavement: diagnosis of South East Asian refugees'. *Social Science and Medicine*, 30: 637–680.

Eitinger, L. (1959) 'The incidence of mental disease among refugees in Norway'. *Journal of Mental Science*, 105: 326–338.

Fernando, S. (1995) (ed.) *Mental Health in a Multi-Ethnic Society*. London: Routledge.

Freed, A. (1988) 'Interviewing through an interpreter'. *Social Work*, July/August, 315–319.

Fuller, K.L. (1993) 'Refugee mental health in Aalborg, Denmark: traumatic stress and cross-cultural treatment issues'. *Nordic Journal of Psychiatry*, 47(4): 251–256.

Furnham, A. and Bochner, S. (1986) *Culture Shock*. London: Routledge.

Gong-Guy, E., Cravens, R.B. and Patterson, T.E. (1991) 'Clinical issues in mental health service delivery to refugees'. *American Psychologist*, 46(6): 642–648.

Gorst-Unsworth, C. and Goldenberg, E. (1998) 'Psychological sequalae of torture and organised violence suffered by refugees from Iraq'. *British Journal of Psychiatry*, 166: 360–367.

Harvey, M. (1984) 'Family therapy with deaf persons. The systemic utilisation of an interpreter'. *Family Process*, 23: 205–213.

Helman, C. (1984) *Culture, Health and Illness*. Bristol: Wright.

Herr, E.L. (1987) 'Cultural diversity from an international perspective'. *Journal of Multicultural Counselling and Development*, 15: 99–109.

Highlen, P.S. (1997) 'MCT theory and implications for organizations/systems'. In D.W. Sue, A.E. Ivey and P.B. Pederson (eds), *A Theory of Multicultural Counselling and Therapy*. Pacific Grove, CA: Brooks/Cole, pp. 65–85.

Hillier, S., Loshak, R., Marks, F. and Rahman, S. (1994) 'An evaluation of child psychiatric services for Bangladeshi parents'. *Journal of Mental Health*, 3: 327–337.

Hitch, P.J. and Rack, P.A. (1980) 'Mental illness among Polish and Russian refugees in Bradford'. *British Journal of Psychiatry*, 137: 206–211.

Hobfoll, S.E., Speilberger, C.D., Folkman, S., Lepper-Green, B., Saranson, I. and Van der Kolk, B. (1991) 'War-related stress addressing the stress of war and other traumatic events'. *American Psychologist*, 46: 848–855.

Hoffman, E. (1989) *Lost in Translation*. London: Minerva.

Home Office (1999) Press and Information Office, Immigration and Nationality Dept, Home Office, Lunar House, Croydon, Surrey, UK. www.homeoffice.gov.uk/rds/immigration1.html

Hough, A. (1991) 'Using complementary or non-verbal therapies with survivors of torture'. Presented at the III International Conference of Centres, Institutions and Individuals concerned with the care of victims of organised violence. Santiago, Chile.

Kelly, P. (1994) 'Integrating systemic and postsystemic approaches to social work practice with refugee families'. *Families in Society*, 75: 541–549.

Kinzie, J.D. and Sack, W. (1991) 'Severely traumatised Cambodian children: research findings and clinical implications'. In F.L. Ahearn and J.L. Athey (eds), *Refugee Children; Theory, Research, and Services* (pp. 92–105). Maryland: Johns Hopkins University Press.

Kleinman, A. (1980) *Patients and Healers in the Context of Culture*. Berkeley: University of California Press.

Kline, F.A. and Spevak, M. (1980) 'Clients evaluate therapists'. *Archive of General Psychiatry*, 31: 113–116.

Kline, F., Acosta, F. and Williams, A. (1980) 'The misunderstood Spanish-speaking patient'. *American Journal of Psychiatry*, 1137: 1530–1533.

Krupinski, J. and Stoller, A. (1965) 'Incidence of mental disorders in Victoria, according to country of birth'. *Medical Journal of Australia*, 2: 265–269.

Lago, C. and Thompson, J. (1996) *Race, Culture and Counselling*. Buckingham: Open University Press.

Landy, D. (1977) (ed.) *Culture, Disease, and Healing: Studies in Medical Anthropology*. New York: Macmillan.

Lau, A. (1985) 'Transcultural issues in family therapy'. *Journal of Family Therapy*, 6: 91–112.

Lavik, N.J., Solberg, O. and Varvin, S. (1997) 'Mental health among refugees. Connection between symptoms, traumatization and exile'. *Tidsskr Nor Laageforen*, 117(25): 36654–36658.

Lewis Fernandez, R. and Kleinman, A. (1995) 'Theoretical, clinical and research issues'. *Psychiatric Clinics of North America*, Sep., 18(3): 433–448.

Light, D. (1992) 'Healing their wounds: Guatemalan refugee women as political activists'. *Women and Therapy*, 13(3): 281–296.

Lopez, A., Boccellari, A. and Hall, K. (1988) 'Post traumatic stress disorder in a central American refugee'. *Hospital and Community Psychiatry*, 39: 1309–1311.

McCallin, M. and Fozzard, S. (1990) *The Impact of Traumatic Events on the Psychological Well-being of Mozambican Refugee Women and Children*. Geneva: International Catholic Child Bureau.

McIvor, R.J. (1994) 'Making the most of interpreters'. *British Journal of Psychiatry*, 165(2): 268.

MacLachlan, M. (1997) *Culture and Health*. Chichester: John Wiley.

Marcos, L. (1979) 'Effects of interpreters on the evaluation of psychopathology in non-English speaking clients'. *Journal of Psychiatry*, 136(2): 171–174.

Mollica, R.F., Wyshak, G. and Lavelle, J. (1987) 'The psychosocial impact of war trauma and torture on Southeast Asian refugees'. *American Journal of Psychiatry*, 144: 1567–1572.

Murphy, H.B.M. (1955) 'Refugee psychoses in Great Britain: admission to mental hospitals. In H.B.M. Murphy (ed.), *Flight and Resettlement*. Paris: UNESCO.

Oberg, K. (1960) 'Cultural shock: adjustment to new cultural environments'. *Practical Anthropology*, 7: 177–182.

Owan, T. (1985) *South East Asian Mental Health: Treatment, Prevention, Services, Training and Research*. Rockville, MD: National Institute for Mental Health.

Racism and Cultural Diversity (2002) European monitoring centre on racism and xenophobia www.eumc.at/publications/media-report/index.htm

Raval, H. (1996) 'A systemic perspective on working with interpreters'. *Clinical Child Psychology and Psychiatry*, 1(1): 29–43.

Refugee Council, Various publications and spokespeople, Press and Information Office, 3, Bondway, London, SW8 1SJ, UK. www.refugeecouncil.org.uk/infocentre/stats/stats007.html

Ressler, E., Boothby, N. and Steinbock, C.J. (1988) *Unaccompanied Children: Care and Protection in Wars, Natural Disasters, and Refugee Movements*. New York: Oxford University Press.

Richman, N. (1998) 'Refugees and asylum-seekers in the west'. In P. Bracken and C. Petty (eds), *Rethinking the Trauma of War*. London: Free Association Books.

Sabin, J.E. (1975) 'Translating despair'. *American Journal of Psychiatry*, 132: 197–199.

Saxthorp, V. and Christiansen, J. (1991) 'Working with refugee families from the Middle East in Denmark'. Presented at the III International Conference of Centres, Institutions and Individuals Concerned with the Care of Victims of Organised Violence and Human Rights, Santiago, Chile.

Shackman, J. (1984) *The Right to be Understood*. London: National Extension College.

Sue, D.W., Carter, R.T., Manuela Casa, J., Fouad, N.A., Ivey, A.E., Jensen, M., La Framboise, T., Manese, J.E., Ponterotto, J.G. and

Vasquez-Nuttal, E. (1988) *Multi-cultural Counseling Competencies. Individual and Organizational Development.* Thousand Oaks, CA: Sage.

Summerfield, D. (1993) 'Addressing human response to war and atrocity: major themes for health workers'. London Medical Foundation for the Care of Victims of Torture.

Summerfield, D. (1998) 'The social experience of war and some issues for the humanitarian field'. In P. Bracken and C. Petty (eds) *Rethinking the Trauma of War* (pp. 9–38). London: Free Association Books.

Torrey, E.F. (1972) *The Mind Game: Witch Doctors and Psychiatrists.* New York: Emerson-Hall.

Trauer, T. (1995) 'Ethnic differences in the utilisation of public psychiatric services in a area of suburban Melbourne'. *Australian & New Zealand Journal of Psychiatry,* 29(4): 615–623.

Tribe, R. (1998) 'If two is company is three a crowd/group? A longitudinal account of a support and clinical supervision group for interpreters'. *Group Work Journal,* 11(3): 139–152.

Tribe, R. (1999a) 'Using interpreters/bicultural workers when working with refugee clients, many who have been tortured'. *British Journal of Medical Psychology,* 72: 567–576.

Tribe, R. (1999b) 'Therapeutic work with refugees living in exile: observations on clinical practice'. *Counselling Psychology Quarterly,* 12(3): 233–243.

Tribe, R. (2002) 'Mental health and refugees'. *Advances In Psychiatric Medicine,* 8(3): 240–248.

Tribe, R. and Sanders, M. (2003) 'Training issues for interpreters'. Chapter 3, this volume.

Tribe, R. and Shackman, J. (1989) 'A way forward: a group for refugee women'. *Group Work Journal,* 2(2): 159–166.

Van der Veer, G. (1992) *Counselling and Therapy with Refugees. Psychological Problems of Victims of War, Torture and Repression.* Chichester: John Wiley.

Venables, M. and Rodriquez, P. (1989) 'A Spanish-speaking psychotherapy group for exiled male victims of torture and political violence'. Presented at the II International Conference of Centres, Institutions and Individuals concerned with the care of victims of organised violence. Costa Rica.

Westwood, M.J. (1990) 'Identification of human problems and methods of help-seeking: a cross cultural study'. Paper presented to the Comparative and International Education Society. Anaheim, California, 29 March to 1 April.

Williams, C. (1989) 'Prevention programs for refugees: an interface for mental health and public health'. *Journal of Primary Prevention,* 10(2): 167–186.

Woodcock, J. (1995) 'Healing rituals with families in exile'. *Journal of Family Therapy*, 17: 397–404.

Yule, W. (1999) (ed.) *Post-Traumatic Stress Disorders, Concepts and Therapy*. Chichester: John Wiley.

Zur, J. (1996) 'From PTSD to voices in context: from an "experience-far" to an "experience-near" understanding of responses to war and atrocity across cultures'. *International Journal of Psychiatry*, 42(4): 305–317.

Chapter 14

Speaking with the silent: addressing issues of disempowerment when working with refugee people[1]

Nimisha Patel

Introduction

The ability to use one's voice in speaking out can be seen as personal power. The opportunity to speak and to use one's voice can be seen as political power. Working with refugee people forces professionals to confront the issue of how we can speak with those who have the capacity to use their voices but who have been systematically persecuted, violated and stripped of their voices, rendering them silent and without personal and political power. Therapeutic work with refugee people often necessitates the use of interpreters to speak on behalf of the refugee person and the therapist. Central to this work is the question 'whose voice matters?'.

This chapter will explore some of the issues of power inherent in therapeutic work with refugee people when using interpreters. It will focus on the question 'who is empowered to speak, for whom and to what end?'. The varying styles of working with interpreters will be identified and suggestions will be made about empowering ways of working with refugee people using interpreters.

Exploring multiple contexts

Refugee people are not a homogenous group, but extremely heterogeneous with diversity in language, culture, political and

---

[1] The commonly used term 'refugees' is considered to be problematic here on the grounds that the legal definition of immigration status is liberally used to label and compartmentalise people who have been forcibly displaced, whilst dehumanising them. Instead, the term 'refugee people' is used to attempt to restore attention to the people whom we burden with legal definitions.

religious affiliations, political histories, experiences of persecution and political violence, and social class, amongst other factors. However, the process of exile, which they all experience, inevitably challenges the very foundations of their relatively stable lives and communities, stripping them of their personal and political power and of their rights to control their lives. Experiences of profound, multiple losses are also common to most refugee people, particularly the loss of the opportunity to use one's voice, in one's own language, to influence one's life in exile. Loss of language refers not to the literal loss of the ability to speak, but to the loss of opportunity to assert and exercise one's rights in exile, particularly when the dominant language is one with which the refugee person is unfamiliar.

The use of political violence, including torture, can also be construed as grossly disempowering in that it systematically violates personal power and attempt to destroy political power. Human rights abuses involving political violence are deliberate and systematic, aiming to intimidate and indoctrinate those who may have tried to exercise their voice and their rights. Indeed, methods of torture are designed to dehumanise, debilitate, disempower and control by terrorising individuals and whole communities, rendering them silent.

Baker's (1992) concept of the 'triple trauma paradigm' further elucidates the nature of exile and its psychosocial implications; the particular impact of torture on refugee people; and what he describes as the further trauma of seeking asylum and refugee status in the UK. He suggests that asylum and immigration legislation and associated procedures in Britain are in themselves torturous, inhuman and degrading, breaching Article 5 of the UN Declaration of Human Rights, 1948. Experiences of individual and institutional racism, which are also human rights abuses, in the country of 'asylum' further marginalise, disempower and silence the already silenced.

It is in this context of human rights abuses world-wide, including Britain, that the offer and use of western psychological models within the therapeutic context with refugee people must be critically viewed. Eurocentric psychological theories and methods are inevitably culturally-bound and biased, which leads to a questioning of their validity in relation to refugee people from non-western backgrounds. Elsewhere, Patel and Fatimilehin (1999) suggest that the blanket imposition and application of inherently biased models to minority ethnic people could be described as secondary colonisation, a process whereby the already marginalised are inadvertently oppressed in the guise of professional 'help'. Similarly, Mollica (1992) points out how current medical and psychological approaches to torture survivors have resulted in a lack of expression by the survivors of their own political, social and personal needs. He argues that 'similar to most oppressed and marginalised populations, the voice of the torture survivor is a whisper (Foucault, 1973)' (Mollica, 1992, p. 25).

The therapeutic context is also fraught with further potentially disempowering and silencing practices when working with interpreters. Interpreters may themselves have refugee backgrounds, with experiences of oppression, political violence and persecution. The therapeutic context offers the interpreter artificial political power, the opportunity to speak, but not always to express one's own perceptions, opinions or voice, but to speak on behalf of the silenced, the refugee client, or on behalf of the therapist. The interpreter's role can be described as facilitating communication, particularly, though not exclusively, using linguistic skills. The interpreter may be positioned as complementary to the process of therapy, though their role results in both the refugee client and the therapist being and feeling dependent on the interpreter. Thus, the interpreter can more accurately be described as holding the most powerful position but paradoxically with the least personal power in the therapeutic context.

Power and the triad of refugee person, interpreter, therapist

The stance of neutrality has been a cornerstone in the majority of western therapeutic models and approaches entrenched in positivist ideologies. Psychological knowledge and activities are thus construed as neutral representations, focusing on individual distress as if it has arisen in and exists in a vacuum, devoid of sociopolitical contexts. The stance of therapeutic neutrality can be criticised for ignoring the historical and socio-political contexts within which human rights abuses have arisen and which are maintained to date, thereby defending and legitimating the ideologies and practices that result in the continued exploitation, oppression and violation of marginalised peoples. It is argued here that any work with refugee people has to be considered and conducted within existing socio-political contexts and that this necessitates that the therapist adopt a non-neutral stance: a stance against human rights abuses. Indeed, Herman (1992), in her work with women survivors of violence, argues that the neutral stance is perhaps an ideal to be striven for, except in the case of moral neutrality. She suggests that 'working with victimised people requires a committed moral stance'. The therapist is called upon to bear witness to a crime. The therapist must affirm a position of 'solidarity' and that 'this involves an understanding of the fundamental injustice of the traumatic experience and the need for resolution that restores some sense of justice' (Herman, 1992, p. 135). As such, the stance of non-neutrality can be interpreted as a political stance against human rights abuses.

Questioning the therapist's political stance in therapy also throws into question the position, stance and role of the interpreter. When the experience of forced exile and possible political violence are conceptualised as the grossest forms of oppression and abuse of power, it becomes imperative that the therapeutic context does not recreate and reinforce the experience of being marginalised, disempowered and silenced. Inevitably, the interpreter is called upon to facilitate communication, not as a neutral linguist, but as an active participant in the struggle against human rights abuses.

The refugee person, the interpreter and the therapist thus engage in a complex web of mutual dependencies, with the explicit aim being to alleviate distress for the refugee person, within a human rights framework. The allegiance against human rights abuses does not preclude other contradictory roles of the therapist, such as the role of assessment and choosing therapeutic interventions, which inadvertently reinforces their own expert position in a way that can further disempower the refugee person and/or the interpreter. Differences between the therapist, the interpreter and the refugee person may become pertinent to the therapeutic process, particularly when issues of power and positioning are considered. Numerous differences may exist between the refugee person, the interpreter and the therapist.

For example, there may exist differences in language, ethnicity, class, gender, age, political and religious beliefs and affiliations (see Figure 14.1). However, such differences are not discrete entities located within each individual concerned, but socially-constructed meanings which determine the nature of the interaction. Thus, difference exists between people and becomes meaningful only in

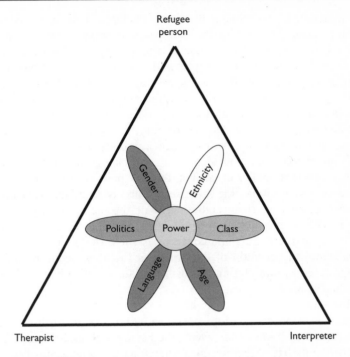

Figure 14.1 Difference and power relations within the refugee person, interpreter, therapist triad

relation to the other. However, meanings attached to particular differences such as in age, are not neutral but inherently socially, historically and culturally bound. The meanings attached to difference in ethnicity may vary depending on cultural, political, historical, or other interpretations all three parties adopt. However, the issue of which meaning is privileged in the therapeutic context depends on who is in a position to define the difference, to give meaning to 'it' and ultimately to exert influence over what action follows. In short, who defines difference and whose interpretation is privileged depends on position and power.

Which voices are silenced, which voices are given a platform and what is spoken are also essentially issues of power. In the therapeutic triad of the refugee person, the interpreter and the therapist, each person is symbolically positioned differently. Ideally the client (refugee person) would be at the apex of any such triad. However, the therapist generally adopts the privileged position at the apex of the triangle, controlling the literal choice of language used in therapy (usually English), the therapeutic context, the choice and use of psychological technologies and perhaps the direction of change. Invariably, the therapist is the driver, the interpreter the vehicle and the client the passenger, each with their explicit positions and roles. However, the interpreter's role in facilitating communication does not mean that they are neutral channels through which therapy proceeds. On the contrary, they are inevitably value-impregnated individuals with their own political, cultural, religious and other proclivities. Their position can change within the triad, either unintentionally, or deliberately, as part of the therapeutic process. For example, the interpreter's ability to adopt particular interpretations of whatever the client or the therapist may say is an inevitable product of their position and role in constructing meaning in the therapeutic context. As such, the interpreter may well adopt the position of the driver, at the apex of the triangle, empowered to interpret and furnish the talk supplied by the client or the therapist.

In stark contrast, there is limited opportunity for the refugee person to choose and adopt positions within the therapeutic context. Their position as the client, the person seeking help, entraps them in a matrix of relationships where they are often compelled to submit to those in relatively more powerful positions: the therapist and the interpreter. Despite any attempts by both the therapist and the interpreter to foster a collaborative, egalitarian relationship, the refugee person is dependent on the therapist in many ways and lacks choice. The refugee person is rarely in a position to choose which language therapy is conducted in, it is usually chosen by the therapist. Occasionally, a therapist may ask the refugee person whether they wish to speak in English if their competency in the English language is sufficient for therapy from the viewpoints of the client and the therapist, or whether they wish to use an interpreter. It is a choice where personal and political power is compromised. This illusion of a choice further obscures the power imbalance inherent in the relationship between the therapist and the refugee person, and can further disempower and silence the already silenced. The refugee person may be asked whether they wish to have an interpreter in a particular language because the refugee person is competent in that language and a relevant interpreter is available. For example, a refugee person from the former Zaire may be asked whether they wish to have a French interpreter, or a French-speaking therapist, rather than a Linghala speaker, with the underlying assumption that the client is competent in French. Here, competency in a language and choice of language may be confused. The refugee person may be competent in French but may not have chosen it as the medium for communication in therapy, perhaps because of associated meanings which regard French as the language of the oppressor, meanings which are historically, culturally and politically significant, but which may be overlooked by the therapist.

In addition, the dependency on an interpreter to make sense of and convey the language used by the refugee person inevitably strips the refugee person of political power, the opportunity to personally define oneself on one's terms and to be more than a passenger or a relatively silent witness to the direction of change. This experience of being disempowered can mirror and replicate previous experiences of being silenced, disempowered, oppressed and violated by those in more privileged positions. For example, the refugee person depends almost entirely on the interpreter to interpret words spoken. Westermeyer (1990) notes that words have specific meanings (cognitive, emotional and symbolic) which require skilful interpretation to transmit connotative and denotative meaning. But this process of interpretation is not neutral in any sense. Interpretation necessitates a process of filtering through the medium of the interpreter, thus all words are coloured by the ideas and value judgements imposed consciously or unconsciously by the interpreter (Haenel, 1997). In essence, the interpreter is empowered to speak on behalf of the refugee person, to create their own language and meaning and to convey that meaning to the therapist in their own words. The refugee person has limited or no choice in this process, particularly whilst they are unfamiliar with the language the therapist has chosen and adopted and the language into which the interpreter interprets the client's words. In adopting a social constructionist stance, Andersen (1992) argues that language is crucial to the constitution of being, that is, language is a way to define oneself and the language used makes the person using it who they are in the moment they use it. By implication, ultimately, the refugee person has limited choice in how they define themselves in language.

There are many challenges for the therapist and the interpreter in therapeutic work. This section has considered one of these challenges: identifying and exploring how one's position endows one with the power to influence the therapeutic process. The following section considers another challenge: exploring and developing more empowering styles of working with refugee people, using interpreters in a way that does not reinforce existing inequalities and experiences of oppression for the refugee person.

Styles of working with interpreters

There are several distinctive, though not mutually exclusive styles that therapists may adopt when working with refugee people using interpreters. These styles, which may overlap or change over time, may require some exploration.

The *constrictive* style is characterised by the therapist assuming an authoritarian stance, positioning themselves at the apex of the triadic relationship between themselves, the client and the interpreter. It is often noticeable in its rigidity and inflexibility in the role and position given to the interpreter. The therapist dictates which position the interpreter adopts without open dialogue and negotiation around the role of the interpreter. The interpreter is expected to do as the therapist does without questioning their stance, and by implication their expert position. This style often treats the interpreter as if they are simply a mouthpiece for the therapist and the client, or what Westermeyer (1990, p. 747) terms a 'word unscrambler', someone 'who merely takes messages from one person and passes them on to the other, without interposing between the patient and the clinician'. The constrictive style also reinforces rigid boundaries and inequalities present in the therapeutic context. The interpreter's interpretation of non-verbal communication or their own values, opinions or viewpoints are not invited by the clinician, and by implication not valued or acknowledged as potential sources of information that may facilitate the therapeutic process, or that may introduce bias or perhaps another layer of meaning which may be of relevance. The client's voice remains silent, except when they are invited by the therapist to speak.

The *vague* or *amorphous* style is characterised by the therapist assuming a stance which does not specify or clarify what the expected position or role of the interpreter is in relation to the client and the therapist. The therapist provides no opportunity to discuss changing roles and positions in the therapeutic process and little explanation or direction is given to the interpreter on how the therapeutic work will proceed, what it will involve and how both can work together. In many ways, the amorphous style leads to a lack of openness, clarity and containment for the interpreter and for the client. The refugee person may experience anxiety and confusion about how they will communicate with the therapist using an interpreter and what they might do if they feel misrepresented, misunderstood or if the process of using an interpreter feels too difficult. This can disempower both the interpreter and the client, leaving both feeling unable to name the difficulties around interpretation or the actual therapeutic context. Interpreters may also be disempowered by not knowing what is expected of them and when, if at all, they are allowed to voice their own opinions or concerns. The 'not knowing' can also serve to silence the silenced. The refugee client may experience the lack of information, clarity, openness and unpredictability as being similar to the experience of systematic state oppression and persecution, where 'not knowing' can lead to persistent arousal, vigilance and anxiety, compounded by not feeling safe or sure about what to expect.

The style of *'human rights workers'* is characterised by the therapist who adopts the stance of 'we're all in this together'. It is a style where the therapist often makes explicit to the refugee person and the interpreter that the therapeutic process will be one characterised by a mutually agreed goal, pursued in solidarity. This can involve the therapist declaring allegiance with the client, against human rights abuses, whilst explicitly or implicitly expecting the interpreter to do the same. It is a style which can be experienced as empowering by the client, and the interpreter, although sometimes it can paradoxically disempower the interpreter who is inadvertently silenced or excluded. For example, the interpreter's indifference, impartiality or discomfort at declaring their political stance can be misinterpreted by the therapist as reluctance to join the political struggle against all human rights abuses, even if there are other factors, such as the interpreter's own differing political, religious, cultural or other affiliations, their own experiences of human rights abuses or their desire to remain detached for personal reasons. Thus, the style of partiality can be empowering to some extent but it can equally be experienced as constrictive, excluding and silencing, particularly by interpreters.

The *judicial* style of working with interpreters is distinctive due to its focused approach with one main aim: to fact-find. This style is more evident and explicit in assessments and more implicit in ongoing therapy. The therapist adopts a somewhat distant, questioning stance, which can be experienced as suspicious and judgmental by the client. The interpreter is expected to interpret whilst making accessible their own hunches and judgements about the refugee client to the therapist. The implicit mission of fact-finding together can involve forming an opinion about the credibility of the client's account on which their asylum claim is based. Fraught with ethical dilemmas, this stance can be experienced as extremely empowering for the interpreter, who is asked at times to go beyond their role in interpreting meaning, to making a judgement about the client. In stark contrast to the elevated position and power ascribed to the interpreter is the position of the refugee person, who is expected to engage in an assessment, perhaps sensing that the interview is conducted in an effort to elucidate 'the truth'. The refugee person can experience this alliance between the therapist and the interpreter as excluding and marginalising, whilst experiencing the fact-finding mission style as an interrogation, perhaps mirroring experiences in detention where interrogation could be accompanied by punishment, usually physical or psychological torture.

The *co-worker* style assumes a collaborative approach that positions the interpreter and the therapist as co-workers in partnership to achieve a mutually agreed aim: to alleviate distress experienced by the refugee client. The co-worker style seeks to create a triad of egalitarian relationships, as far as is possible, between the interpreter, therapist and the refugee client. Therapeutic agendas are openly negotiated, issues of power are acknowledged and explored and the opinions of the interpreter are invited, heard and valued by the therapist. There is a commitment to openness and transparency within clearly articulated and flexible boundaries. This style can be experienced as immensely empowering for both the interpreter and the refugee client and enable a humanitarian, respectful approach to be developed. However, there is a danger in assuming that a co-worker style somehow removes the power imbalance inherent in the triad within the therapeutic context. In fact, the therapist remains the main driver with the interpreter as a co-driver who is sometimes allowed to drive, using their own expertise and knowledge.

Throughout the therapeutic process, the client is encouraged by the therapist and the interpreter to drive. The therapist may facilitate the development of the client's ability to use their voice and attempt to create opportunities for the client to exercise their voice in making choices, shaping meaning and controlling the pace and direction of change. However, the co-worker style may give rise to the illusion of equality and of power balance, which is arguably impossible within the context of therapy where there are inherent inequalities and power relations, maintained by the very act of therapy. Westermeyer (1990, p. 747) indicates that the roles of the interpreter, the clinician and the client are dissimilar in terms of professional, legal or symbolic status, arguing that 'although the patient can "hire or fire" the other two, there exists the imposing physical fact of two staff against one patient . . . the clinician is [also] legally and ethically in charge of the interpreter and the interview process, a fact that must be appreciated by the interpreter'.

The *colonial* style is perhaps the most subtle and difficult to explore as a style because of its covert and perhaps unintentional racism. It is a style which interpreters can often be acutely aware of but which they feel particularly disempowered to name or to challenge. The therapist assumes the position of the rescuer, the bountiful benefactor and bestower of kindness, goodness and technology to alleviate the distress experienced by the refugee client. The interpreter is a facilitator in this process, an implied ally of the therapist but also positioned sometimes as a compatriot and as a potential ally to the refugee client. This style, like other styles, has implicit functions, for example, possibly serving the function of appeasing the conscience of the therapist who may themselves feel disempowered and helpless in the face of overwhelming adversity experienced by the refugee client, and perhaps the interpreter. The therapist is empowered to deliver a technology or to provide material, social, medical or emotional assistance. The interpreter can be disempowered by being expected to interpret for a therapist, and in a way which they and the refugee client experience as patronising and colonialist, yet feel unable to challenge. The refugee client may experience a conflict between seeking alliance with the interpreter or in distancing themselves from the interpreter and the therapist from embarrassment, shame, anger or resentment. Their position as refugee people in exile commonly means they have nothing or very little, they may have experienced multiple losses, persecution and political violence, been robbed of their dignity and their emotional, social, spiritual and physical health, and they may exist in a depleted social world, subjected to hostility, suspicion and racism within the receiving country. The offer of support cannot be easily rejected when one is silenced and impoverished in exile, thus entrapping the refugee person in a web of inequalities, imbalanced relationships and of mutual debt and obligation. The colonial style can be profoundly disempowering for both the interpreter and client, regardless of the benevolent intentions of the therapist.

In exploring these differing styles, therapists could begin to develop more empowering ways of working with interpreters to facilitate the therapeutic process. Some of the key features of empowering ways of working with interpreters are considered in the following section.

Challenging the silence

To speak with the silenced, using interpreters, can be a professional and personal challenge for the therapist and the interpreter. As potential tools in the therapeutic process both the interpreter and the therapist are required to pay attention to the areas of their practice which further silence the silenced. Thus, challenging this silence becomes a collaborative enterprise involving reflexivity, openness and professional maturity. Central to this process have to be the principles of empowerment, non-exploitation, respect, humanitarianism and accountability. All require that ultimately, the safety and welfare of the client are primary aims.

Political persecution and exile result in the violation of every kind of boundary crucial to well-being. Geographical boundaries are challenged, the concept of home and homeland rendered incomprehensible or an unachievable ideal, linguistic boundaries stretched, distorted, destroyed, family and other social networks fragmented, communities shattered and personal physical, spiritual and emotional boundaries subjected to brutal assaults. Most refugee people have experienced a catalogue of assaults on, and challenges to, every personal and social boundary known to them. Those who have experienced torture will also have encountered the deliberate, systematic and state-sanctioned violation of human rights, the basic boundaries of humanity.

The purposes of torture are complex yet consistent: to create physical and psychological debility; and to destroy personal and social resistance. As such, torture involves the rupture of interpersonal attachments, which Saporta and van der Kolk (1992) suggest leads to traumatic bonding where survivors attempt to maintain attachment bonds to regain a state of psychological and physiological calm, by forming strong emotional ties with their torturers. It is this relationship which can be recreated in the therapeutic context with the interpreter and the therapist, who may unwittingly further disempower the refugee client by neglecting to consider the significance of the context within which previous attachments and boundaries have been violated and of the therapeutic context within which new bonds are formed.

Establishing safety and a non-exploitative and non-abusive environment requires that both the therapist and the interpreter are rigorous in developing professional boundaries and in respecting the significance of the refugee client's attachments to them. Time-keeping is an example of how the therapist's failure to explain the significance of time-keeping and boundaries to the interpreter can lead to the therapist being consistent and punctual, whilst the interpreter may not be, resulting in the abuse of the refugee client.

In reviewing experimental models relevant to refugee people who have been tortured, Basoglu and Mineka (1992) suggest that the concepts of control and prediction are crucial to the therapeutic process. The unpredictability of events surrounding exile, and particularly torture, can result in a chronic state of fear. Torture survivors have often experienced prolonged periods of unpredictable stress, not knowing when the next torture session will begin, when the sounds of footsteps outside one's cell signals more torture, or not knowing what they will be subjected to next. Basoglu and Mineka (1992) indicate that providing predictability by giving certain types of information about the nature of traumatic stimuli to be encountered can reduce stress for some people, particularly for 'high monitors', those who prefer to cope with stressful experiences by monitoring the details of what is happening (see Miller, 1980, 1989).

In the therapeutic process, a context laden with potentially stressful stimuli, one needs to consider how some stimuli could remind the client of previous experiences of torture. Inevitably, the interpreter and the therapist become collaborators in the therapeutic process and in providing predictability for the client, as far as is possible, they could minimise the distress encountered by the client. It is often enormously helpful to the client if they are informed in advance of the fact that an interpreter will be present, particularly on first appointments. Ensuring predictability can also require both the therapist and the interpreter to carefully consider together how best to introduce the topic of working therapeutically with an interpreter. The client needs to be informed of what the role of the interpreter is, how therapeutic sessions will be conducted with interpreters, the name of the interpreter, and sometimes the client may ask what the ethnic, geographical or cultural background of the interpreter is for fear of further retribution if the interpreter is from an opposing political or ethnic group, perhaps one from which the client has experienced persecution or violence. The not knowing can contribute to increased fear, suspicion and mistrust, which can be further compounded by the indifference or unwillingness on the part of the therapist and the interpreter to make explicit their roles or backgrounds. Discussion of these issues and preparation between the therapist and interpreter can facilitate the establishment of a safe, therapeutic environment, without necessarily involving self-disclosure. The therapist and interpreter can also prepare by agreeing which information to provide the client with on commencing therapy. For example, the nature and purpose of therapy, the approach to be adopted, the procedure for making appointments, managing cancellations, making a complaint or providing feedback to the therapist, interpreter or an independent person about the service received.

Uncontrollability is also a crucial concept in developing more empowering ways of working with refugee clients using interpreters. Uncontrollability plays an important role in the aetiology and maintenance of fear and anxiety (Mineka and Kelly, 1989). In reviewing the literature in this area, Basoglu and Mineka (1992) conclude that once fear or anxiety has been acquired, gaining experience with control over the source of anxiety and therapeutic interventions aimed at increasing perception of control can be beneficial in its reduction.

Where experiences of exile and torture have increased the refugee person's perception of and actual uncontrollability in relation to their own personal selves and to their environment, therapists and interpreters can collaborate in maximising the perception of and actual control afforded to the client; for example, respecting the person's autonomy, their personal and political power in using their voices, in making choices and in effecting change. Informed consent to working with an interpreter becomes as important as informed consent to engaging in a therapeutic encounter or process. The therapist and interpreter may need to negotiate how to enable the refugee client to assert their viewpoints and make choices, for example, choosing the gender of the interpreter, or choosing the language in which therapy can proceed. A female refugee client with experiences of gender-based persecution and violence may not know that she can choose to have a female interpreter, nor may she feel able to declare this preference to the therapist for fear of being dismissed, punished, ignored or ridiculed, or she may not be literally able to communicate this to the therapist when she has to rely on a male interpreter, perhaps from her own cultural background, to speak on her behalf. Creating opportunities to choose requires that both the therapist and the interpreter jointly invite and endorse choices made by the client and communicate that the therapeutic process is a journey that requires that all parties take turns to drive, and thus sanctioning the client assuming control.

However, creating opportunities for the client to assume control is insufficient in itself, particularly when the experience of torture has resulted in its intended outcome: the loss of control and the increase in unpredictability. The therapeutic process in itself is likely to be insufficient to compensate for the lack of predictable, safe social networks or to counteract the effects of continued unpredictable and uncontrollable experiences in society, including experiences of homelessness, poverty, destitution and racism. Sometimes, the interpreter can become a figure on whom the client relies and entrusts with the hope that the interpreter can help them in other areas, such as with their housing or medical needs. The therapist's role is to enable the interpreter to discuss these demands and dilemmas they experience in relation to the client, within the therapeutic context, so as not to overload and disempower the interpreter nor leave them carrying the responsibility of assuming control over the client's life or of restoring control to the client.

Interpreters are also often implicitly or explicitly expected to assume many other responsibilities within the therapeutic context. The responsibility of communicating culturally-specific verbal or non-verbal communication to the therapist and to the client is one example. The interpreter is invariably responsible for interpreting meanings in communication from both the client and the therapist and for conveying that meaning to the relevant other in a way which is culturally comprehensible. Shackman (1984) notes that confusion and misunderstanding can result from a lack of familiarity with cultural beliefs and norms, information which she argues the interpreter could convey to the professional. Similarly, Raval (1996) suggests that interpreters' cultural understanding of the client's culture can make accessible services which may not have otherwise been possible. The responsibility of being a culture-broker has attached additional burdens and possible pitfalls for the interpreter.

The interpreter can be endowed with the responsibility of recognising, interpreting and communicating the nuances of culturally-shaped behaviours and beliefs. Whilst being given a respectable position as a driver in the therapeutic context, the interpreter can feel obliged to offer 'cultural interpretations', thus being responsible for speaking on behalf of the client and their own perception of and relationship to their culture. As Wright (1998) reminds us, 'culture' is a dynamic concept, always negotiable and in a process of contestation and transformation. What is particularly significant is that interpreters are positioned such in relation to the client that they are asked to assume the power to define 'culture' as it means to the client. The burden of the expert position can prevent them from freely exploring and communicating the historical, political and economic factors that have shaped their own interpretations of the culture in question. A middle class, educated man from an urban setting does not necessarily have the same experience nor understanding of culture that a female client from a rural background within the same country might.

The addition of variables of ethnicity, religion, class, political background, age and gender weave many other layers of meaning with culture, meanings which can differ for both the interpreter and the client. Thus, the interpreter as a culture-broker, or a bi-cultural colleague, is a role fraught with contradictions, pitfalls and potential for gross misinterpretations. Whilst the interpreter cannot be expected to represent all aspects, experiences and interpretations of a given culture, their points of view can be a valid addition to the construction of meaning. However, this requires the therapist to discuss and explore the cultural interpretations with the interpreter, before and after sessions, but most importantly, also during therapeutic sessions, with the client. Transparency and a willingness to plead ignorance and bias are necessary prerequisites for empowering both client and interpreter, thus creating opportunities to reflect on the process by which culture is made meaningful in relation to each specific client. This further demands that culture and culturally-shaped meanings are not simply explored as if culture is that which is possessed by only the client and the interpreter, but also by the therapist. The culturally-shaped assumptions and values held by the therapist and implicit in the psychological models and methods employed should therefore become open to discussion, scrutiny and challenge by both the client and the interpreter.

Interpreters can be extremely valuable assets to the therapeutic process, a process which necessitates all parties being active participants in the therapeutic system. Haenal (1997) draws attention to the ways in which interpreters can experience the refugee client's transference as well as develop their own countertransference reactions. For example, interpreters may experience profound guilt if they had somehow escaped the brutalities experienced by the client in their homeland; or they may develop feelings of extreme helplessness, powerlessness and anxiety, which may be very relevant in the context of therapeutic work with a client whose predicament, management and expression of their feelings are such that all witnesses, including the therapist, feel very powerless. Such information is crucial to the therapeutic process and where the interpreter experiences much of what the therapist might ordinarily experience, it becomes imperative that the therapist is able to provide the interpreter with support and space to discuss these feelings in relation to the client. Whilst the therapist cannot assume a therapeutic role with the interpreter, it is also an ethical obligation and a professional responsibility to ensure that interpreters are provided with or have access to support, and supervision if appropriate, outside the context of their work with the client and the therapist in question.

Haenel (1997) posits that countertransferential reactions in both the therapist and the client are signs that they have become too close empathically to the client. Thus, the interpreter may suffer from 'vicarious traumatisation', experiencing the same difficulties as the client. He suggests that post-session discussion and Balint[2] or supervision groups for interpreters would be helpful for these reasons. Others have also reiterated the importance of providing

---

[2] Haenal (1997, p. 71) describes Balint groups (developed by Michael Balint, 1896–1970) as working groups where professional helpers discuss their experiences with clients in regular sessions facilitated by a group leader to 'make evident the thoughts, feelings and value judgements of helpers towards their clients, to prevent enmeshment and to provide an anxiety-free communication with their clients'.

support and supervision groups for interpreters working with refugees (e.g. Tribe, 1998). However, this does not preclude additional discussions between the therapist and the interpreter, particularly when the interpreter becomes distressed during or after a particular session. The therapist must be careful not to pathologise the interpreter or their distress, nor exclude or minimise their experience. Empowering practice requires that the therapist is non-exploitative and not oppressive, not just towards the client, but also towards the interpreter.

In conclusion, speaking for the silenced is undoubtedly and inevitably a disempowering act, disempowering those we seek to empower and whose voices we wish to amplify. The task for therapists is to continually develop reflexivity and create ways to work with interpreters which do not reinforce human rights violations by further stripping refugee clients of their personal and political power to influence their lives. The task for interpreters is to engage in a creative and demanding process with the paramount aim of allowing the whispers of the silenced to be heard.

Acknowledgements

Appreciation is extended to all the interpreters I have worked with over the years and who have influenced my thinking and practice. In particular, I would like to thank Berivan Dosky, Agostinho Mbala and Hasan Gok who have helped me enormously in understanding the complexity of working with refugee people, using interpreters.

References

Andersen, T. (1992) 'Reflections on reflecting, with families'. In S. McNamee and K. Gergen (eds), *Therapy as Social Construction*. London: Sage.
Baker, R. (1992) 'Psychosocial consequences for tortured refugees seeking asylum and refugee status in Europe'. In M. Basoglu (ed.), *Torture and its Consequences, Current Treatment Appendices*. Cambridge: Cambridge University Press.
Basoglu, M. and Mineka, S. (1992) 'The role of uncontrollable and unpredictable stress in post-traumatic stress responses in torture survivors'. In M. Basoglu (ed.), *Torture and its Consequences, Current Treatment Approaches*. Cambridge: Cambridge University Press.

Foucault, M. (1973) *Madness and Civilisation: Its History of Insanity in the Age of Reason*. New York: Random House.

Haenel, F. (1997) 'Aspects and problems associated with the use of interpreters in psychotherapy of victims of torture'. *Torture*, 7(3): 68–71.

Herman, J. (1992) *Trauma and Recovery, from Domestic Abuse to Political Terror*. London: Pandora.

Miller, S. (1980) 'Why having control reduces stress: if I can stop the roller coaster I don't want to get off'. In M. Seligman and J. Garber (eds), *Human Helplessness: Theory and Applications*. New York: Academic Press.

Miller, S. (1989) 'Information, coping and control in patients undergoing surgery and stressful medical procedures'. In A. Steptoe and A. Appels (eds), *Stress, Personal Control and Health*. Chichester: John Wiley.

Mineka, S. and Kelly, K. (1989) 'The relationship between anxiety, lack of control and loss of control'. In A. Steptoe and A. Appels (eds), *Stress, Personal Control and Health*. Chichester: John Wiley.

Mollica, R. (1992) 'The prevention of torture and the clinical care of survivors: a field in need of a new science'. In M. Basoglu (ed.), *Torture and its Consequences, Current Treatment Approaches*. Cambridge: Cambridge University Press.

Patel, N. and Fatimilehin, I. (1999) 'Racism and mental health'. In C. Newnes, G. Holmes and C. Dunn (eds), *This is Madness. A Critical Look at Psychiatry and the Future of Mental Health Services*. Ross-on-Wye: PCCS.

Raval, H. (1996) 'A systemic perspective on working with interpreters'. *Clinical Child Psychology and Psychiatry*, 1(1): 29–43.

Saporta, J. and van der Kolk, B. (1992) 'Psychobiological consequences of severe trauma'. In M. Basoglu (ed.), *Torture and its Consequences, Current Treatment Approaches*. Cambridge: Cambridge University Press.

Shackman, J. (1984) *The Right to be Understood. A Handbook on Working with, Employing and Training Community Interpreters*. Cambridge: National Extension College.

Tribe, R. (1998) 'If two is company is three a crowd/group? A longitudinal account of a support and clinical supervision group for interpreters'. *Group Work Journal*, 11(3): 139–152.

Westermeyer, J. (1990) 'Working with an interpreter in psychiatric assessment and treatment'. *Journal of Nervous and Mental Disease*, 178(12): 745–749.

Wright, S. (1998) 'The politicisation of "culture"'. *Anthropology Today*, 14(1): 7–15.

Chapter 15

Narratives of translating–interpreting with refugees: the subjugation of individual discourses

Renos K. Papadopoulos

The poetic moves in life

'The poet moves from life to language. The translator moves from language to life; both, like the immigrant, try to identify the invisible, what's between the lines, the mysterious implications'. In this telling passage, from her novel *Fugitive Pieces* (1996, p. 109), Anne Michaels attempts to convey the dynamics involved in translating. Although she is addressing here the specific theme of translation in poetry, nevertheless, this passage offers two important insights which are of wider relevance to translation in general: these are the reciprocal movement from 'life' to 'language', and the similarities between translation and the 'immigrant' condition.

The translator's task, according to Michaels, is to redirect and reverse the creative process of the poet by reconnecting the poem back to the body of life-experiences, out of which the poet had originally moulded the poem. This reconnection with life implies that the translator is capable of conducting this reverse operation on the basis of a shared body of experiences with the poet. In other words, it is implied that the translator is intimately familiar with the poet's life-experiences and that they also share other relevant sensitivities. This is a sound understanding of the translation process and it can be applied to other forms of translation, including translating in therapeutic interventions when clients and therapists do not speak the same language and, therefore, they require the services of specialist interpreters.

However, despite its simple formulation and evident truth, this understanding is limited because it ignores many other aspects of translation which are of equal importance to the interaction between 'life' and 'language'. To begin with, are life and language so antithetical; are they mutually exclusive? Then, is it correct to accept that the poem is a dried out formula without any life of its own? Life, surely, is not only present as the source of the poem; the poem itself, as well as its translation, have their own life and they can become sources of inspiration as much as life itself can. Yet, undeniably, the oppositionality between 'life' and 'language' makes sense; there is a world of 'words' as distinct from the world of 'deeds'. Thus, the relationship between 'life' and 'language' remains a complex one. This is why Michaels introduces the second aspect of translation when she likens both the poet and translator to the immigrant. The image of immigrant introduces to this intricate process the otherness, strangeness, unknownness, 'the invisible, . . . the mysterious implications'. Poets, translators and immigrants find themselves in new territories where they have to maintain a workable balance between the old and the new, the security of the familiar and the excitement of the unfamiliar, and to weigh up the risks between remaining rigid or losing their sense of proportion; it is not easy to survive in a new country, with all the debilitating perils and promising opportunities.

Immediately preceding the passage quoted above, Michaels states that 'Translation is a kind of transubstantiation; one poem becomes another' (1996, p.109). Undoubtedly, there is something mysterious about 'transubstantiation', the change from one substance to another. Does the 'form' change but the 'substance' remain the same? What is the relationship between the two? What is the context within which these changes take place? If this new passage from Michaels raises additional questions, at least it submits one important affirmation – that the translated poem is another poem in its own right, which requires to be respected as such. Thus, although there is a temptation to see a linear sequence of increasing distance from life to the poem and then from the poem to its translation, this passage helps us to appreciate that such a simplification would be erroneous. Accordingly, the original interaction between life and language needs to be enlarged to include the poem and its translation. This means that we now have a network of interactions among these four elements instead of the oppositionality of the primary two. Needless to say, there is a host of additional factors involved in this process such as the personalities of the poet and the translator as well as their gender, historical times, locations, socio-economic, political and religious background, to name but a few.

These considerations and questions about translation in poetry can equally be applied to the work of interpreters in mental health. Nobody would argue against the assertion that the task of interpreters, in this context, is to endeavour to provide as accurate translations as possible of what the clients say to their therapists. Nevertheless, the situation is fairly complex and it would be beneficial to reflect on issues pertaining to translation and interpretation in wider contexts.

Translation and interpretation

The standard definitions of translation and interpretation provide us with a slight difference between them, although they are often used in a synonymous way. The Oxford English Dictionary defines the verb 'translate' as 'express the sense of (word, sentence, speech, book, poem, etc. . . .) in or into another language; in or to another form of representation'; also, it refers to 'move from one person, place or condition to another'. The Latin 'translatio' means 'transferring, handing over'; 'latio' means 'bringing' and 'trans-latio' would be to bring across, to transfer. The connotation is that of a simple transfer from one locus to another without changes. Interpretation, on the other hand, has a deeper meaning. The Oxford English Dictionary defines 'interpret' as 'expound the meaning of; make out the meaning of; bring out the meaning of; render, by artistic representation or performance; explain, understand'. The usual way that the Latin 'interpretatio' is translated is as 'explanation' and its etymological root 'pretium' means 'worth, value, price'. Thus, interpretation has, unmistakably, an additional meaning over and above the simple transfer: it contains elements of evaluation, explanation and understanding. This signifies that meaning in translation is moved from one context to another on what could be conceived as a horizontal plane, whereas in interpretation, meaning acquires an additional quality (evaluative or explaining) and therefore, it could be understood that the movement takes place along a vertical axis. Thus, interpretation is often seen as offering a 'deeper' or 'higher' meaning than that which a mere translation affords.

The view that translation is a horizontal move, transferring meaning in an intact way, without additions or subtractions, evaluation or interpretation seems to represent a theoretical ideal. In practice, it is impossible to transfer meaning 'from one person, place or condition to another' without changes taking place. Language theorists have identified various conditions that need to be met in order to have a perfect translation. Ogden and Richards, for example, in their classic study on *The Meaning of Meaning*, argued that there are 'several quite intelligible reasons' ([1923] 1949, p. 228) that contribute to the success or failure of translation. Firstly, with reference to symbolic use of words, translation is possible 'if in the two vocabularies similar symbolic distinctions have been developed' (p.228); if this is not the case, then 'new symbols will be required'. However,

> the more emotive functions are involved the less easy will be the task of blending several of these [symbols] in the two vocabularies. And further, the greater the use made in the original of the direct effects of words through rhythm, vowel-quality, etc., the more difficult will it be to secure similar effects in the same way in a different sound-medium. Thus some equivalent method has to be introduced, and this tends to disturb the other functions so that what is called the 'success' of a translation is often due chiefly to its own intrinsic merits.
> (Ogden and Richards, [1923] 1949, p. 229)

This means that although one may be able to distinguish several clear and 'intelligible' factors contributing to a successful translation, their implementation creates difficulties such as the horizontal transfer from one language to another of various complex elements, e.g. symbols, emotion, rhythm.

It is useful to be reminded that, in linguistics, three types of translation are usually distinguished: intra-lingual translation, which involves using different words from the same language to paraphrase a meaning; inter-lingual translation, which renders meaning from one language to another; and 'intersemiotic translation' (Jakobson, 1971), which recodes signs from one sign system to another, e.g. verbal to non-verbal. Explaining further the third type of translation, Marshall Edelson clarified that, 'Translation need not involve two natural languages but may involve translation from one kind of semiotic system to another, for example, from image to language' (1975, p.40). Once it is appreciated that translation encompasses all these types of activities, it is possible to accept that it is much closer to interpretation than traditional definitions suggest.

George Steiner (1975, p.45) conceded that, in effect, every kind of translation involves a degree of interpretation. Moreover, he emphasised that 'any model of communication is at the same time a model of trans-lation, of a vertical or horizontal transfer of significance' and further clarified that 'No two historical epochs, no two social classes, no two localities use words and syntax to signify exactly the same things, to send identical signals of valuation and inference. Neither do two human beings'. In other words, every kind of communication and understanding involves a degree of both translation and interpretation. Aptly, the title of the chapter where he develops these ideas is entitled 'Understanding as translation'. Understanding entails an act of transferring meaning from one context to another and this amounts to translation. In this way, Steiner asserted that translation from one language to another (inter-lingual translation) consists of the same processes which are included in our attempt to understand our own language (intra-lingual translation):

> The model 'sender to receiver' which represents any semio-logical and semantic process is ontologically equivalent to the model 'source-language to receptor-language' used in the theory of [inter-lingual] translation. In both schemes there is 'in the middle' an operation of interpretative decipherment, an encoding–decoding function or synapse.
>
> (Steiner, 1975, p. 47)

In so far as this 'interpretative decipherment', this 'synapse' which connects the two parts of a communication dyad is common to all types of translation, Steiner declared that 'in short: inside or between languages, human communication equals translation' (p.47).

These are important considerations which affect the way we approach inter-lingual translation, in general, and in mental health settings, in particular. We are now able to appreciate that the difficulties interpreters face in these contexts are not limited to those concerning translating inter-lingually but also intra-lingually and inter-semiotically. Indeed, their job involves interpretative decipherment across several sign systems and contexts; these include linguistic, cultural, socio-political, historical, professional, legal, emotional, etc.

Post-traumatic narratives and interpreting time sequences

Translation inter-lingually and inter-semiotically has striking similarities with interpretation in the psychotherapeutic process in so far as all entail transfer of meaning from one context to another; similarities between translation and psychotherapy have been identified by many authors, each emphasising different aspects (e.g. Adams, 1992; Cheshire, 1975; Dallos, 1997; de Certeau, 1986; Edelson, 1975; Flanders, 1993; Fromm, 1951; Kugler, 1982; Maffei, 1986; Mahony, 1987; Muller, 1996; Rimmon-Kenan, 1987; Siegelman, 1990). Essentially, the therapist is called upon to translate the language of symptoms to another system which is comprehensible to the patient. Moreover, it is accepted that psychotherapy goes beyond a mere horizontal translation, as it is also expected to bring about an actual transformation in the patient. This means that the translation in therapy must include additional elements, which encourage such shifts in the patients that enable them to move into different modes of being. Such shifts are accounted for by different psychotherapeutic systems in different ways, e.g. rendering unconscious motives conscious (psychoanalytic), expanding their epistemology (systemic), actualising their being (humanistic), advancing their individuation process (Jungian).

One of the themes that usually dominates the therapeutic work with refugees is that of trauma. Undeniably, a lot of refugees are exposed to traumatic experiences and it is appropriate that part of the therapeutic work with them should involve addressing their trauma. However, the widespread and indiscriminate use of the diagnosis of Post-Traumatic Stress Disorder (PTSD), along with the various set therapeutic interventions which purport to treat it, create many difficulties. Although a detailed examination and a critique of PTSD with reference to refugee work is beyond the scope of this chapter (for this see Bracken, 1998; Bracken and Petty, 1998; Friedman and Jaranson, 1994; Marsella, 1996a, 1996b; Papadopoulos, 1997, 1998; Papadopoulos and Hildebrand, 1997; Richman, 1998), a discussion concerning its relation to the translating issues is indicated.

Often practitioners fall into the trap of focusing too much on the original trauma experienced by a refugee client, as this is one area which seems to have an 'objective and tangible' quality about it.

Ignatieff (1999) warns practitioners not to be seduced and become fascinated with the original trauma at the expense of other important areas that the client may wish to address with the practitioner. Focusing too exclusively on the original events or 'dominant trauma discourse' is unhelpful and may preclude accessing alternative stories and strengths that a client may hold.

Conceptualising trauma as consisting primarily of a before and after phase has the effect of subjugating other important stories that a person may hold about him or herself. The process of coming through trauma is a complex one that is dependent on many other factors such as the person's prior life experiences and emotional (and material) resources, consequent life events, fears held by the person, and individual narratives (old and new narratives) that develop. For many people life experiences following the original 'traumatic event' may be far more negative than the original event. For example, adapting to new types of prejudices and discriminations in a host country may be far more emotionally draining than continuing to live in a hostile but familiar environment. Also, given that individuals construct their own unique life stories and meanings about their experiences, it is not surprising that each person will react differently to what may seem at face value to be similar life experiences. In a similar way to how people's stories change over time and circumstances, it is important to note that language and meaning too change over time. The process of translation has to take this into account if the interpretation is to retain meaning.

When different difference matters

Living in a new country with all its pressures and necessary adjustments is not easy, especially when many people from the host country may appear to be uncaring or unable to understand the life experiences that a refugee person has undergone. In such circumstances people new to a country may form intentionally or spontaneously what may be called 'storied communities' (Papado-poulos, 1996b). Such communities can serve the positive function of fostering resilience and providing a 'secure base' for those in it (Bowlby, [1973] 1985, 1988). Also, people usually live within numerous contexts at the same time (Bateson, [1969] 1972). The tensions associated with the latter can create either the potential for resilience to be fostered, or produce setting conditions that are not conducive to psychological well-being.

Interpreters may or may not be members of particular community groups, and consideration may need to be given to the advantages and disadvantages associated with this connection or lack of, when booking an interpreter to work with a particular client. Sharing a community context may help with the process of engaging with a client, as will connections available through other attributes such as language, country of origin, gender, ethnicity, religion, etc. On other occasions specific differences may become more prominent, negating the connections available through shared attributes. For example, similarities of gender, country of origin, religion may no longer be enough to sustain engagement with a client where perhaps issues of political affiliation become apparent in the work making it difficult for the client to continue with the same interpreter because of their differences. It is often difficult to predict at the outset which attributes, or level of matching of the interpreter with a client, are likely to facilitate or hinder engagement with a client, particularly when different factors may become more prominent or significant for the client at different points in time.

Dramatis personae

What is usually emphasised in most texts about interpreters in mental health contexts are the accuracy of their translation and their own feelings as witnesses to a drama where they are assumed to play a rather peripheral role (Pentz-Moller et al, 1988; Putsch, 1985; Sabin, 1975; van der Veer, 1998). Yet, in so far as interpreters are present in the therapy room they could be considered as participants of this tripartite interaction. At the extreme end of the spectrum there is even the view that if the sole role of the interpreter is to enable a smooth linguistic communication between the therapist and the refugee and if there were also issues of confidentiality at stake, then the interpreter should not even be physically present in the therapeutic session. Commenting about such circumstances, van der Veer advocates the following:

> One way of maintaining the client's anonymity, and thereby increasing the chance he will discuss his problems openly, is to use a loudspeaker telephone and the services of external

interpreters. Then the interpreter need not meet the refugee personally; he does not know what he looks like and need not even know his name. The disadvantage of this method is that gestures and other non-verbal aspects of communication are lost.

(Van der Veer, 1998, p. 83)

Is it only the non-verbal aspects of the communication that are lost? Is a disembodied voice better than the presence of a human being who can be in an acknowledged position of interaction with the refugee and the therapist?

Ordinarily, therapeutic interaction is between a therapist and a patient. However, when an interpreter is present it is not possible to pretend that he/she is not there. Systemic family therapists have long been interested in the composition of therapeutic systems and have found ways of integrating in the therapeutic process observers to whom they assigned varied roles – these range from sitting behind the screen of the one-way mirror to being present in the room; from commenting at the end of the session, to interrupting the session in order to offer their feedback. Creative ways have been devised to enable feedback from such additional parties to the therapeutic dyad to be integrated within the therapeutic process; these ways include ideas such as the 'Greek chorus' (Papp, 1980) and the 'reflecting team' (Andersen, 1987; 1992). Essentially, systemic therapists accepted that it is not possible to be a fly on the wall and that anybody present in the room (or even behind the screen) is a member of the therapeutic system. As a feeling, reacting, and reflecting person the interpreter cannot be a mere translating device.

Another perspective on the presence of the interpreter in the therapeutic system can be developed on the basis of the discussion on translation above. The logical oppositionality between 'life' and 'language' was broken up by the inclusion of other elements such as the 'poem' and its 'translation'. It is easy to think that what is involved in writing a poem is a (horizontal) translation of a given set of life experiences into a language system and then in translation the translator replaces one language system with another, whilst retaining the same referential basis. Although such a simplistic view is tempting, we all know that language and the poem have their own 'independent' lives and that it is not a question of a mere translation from life to a poem and from one language to another. The linear opposition between 'life experience' and its 'verbal expression' (or to use the semiotic terms: from the signified to the signifier), which appeals to common sense, breaks down under closer scrutiny. As Steiner observed, the simple model of 'sender to receiver' always includes the 'interpretative decipherment', that crucial 'synapse' in the middle which breaks the tyranny of linear and dual oppositionality. The 'language' of life is different from the language of the poem and at the same time they are interrelated; the process of writing a poem does not involve a mere horizontal transfer of meaning from one discrete system to another. Language shapes our experiences as well as our experiences shape our language. The relationship is not that of a linear opposition but that of a circular or reflexive co-construction. The one defines the other.

Thus, 'Translation is . . . necessarily a *critical* activity, a mode of *deconstruction*, that is, the undoing of an illusory historical perception or understanding by bearing witness to what the 'perception' or the 'understanding' precisely fails to see or fails to witness' (Felman and Laub, 1992, p. 160). This means that translation necessarily involves not only interpretation but also some kind of correction, a critical stance, an articulation of what the text does not say explicitly, although it is implied (if we cared to 'deconstruct' it) in the way the text was constructed. Translation needs to adjust the 'original' meaning because it is 'deficient' and 'deceptive', and to locate the meaning in its context. The 'original' meaning is flawed and illusory and 'fails to witness' because by remaining focused on its subject matter it fails to address itself in the process. For example, when refugees talk in therapy about their feelings and reactions during the period of the 'original trauma' (i.e., the sub-phase of the devastating events), they are not likely also to offer any self-reflexive comments; e.g. on what made them choose the words and imagery in their narrative, or on their unconscious expectations about the impact their narrative would have on their interpreter and therapist, or on the wider impact on the formulation of their story by the dominant discourse (i.e. of the tyranny of the 'post'). As therapists, if our concerns were to be limited to how accurately the refugees conveyed in words what they had indeed experienced at the time (i.e. whether they selected the best signifier to accurately reflect the signified), we would ignore all the other considerations which are also included in their statements but not explicitly uttered by them. Deconstruction is the term introduced by 'post-structuralists' (e.g. Derrida, 1978; 1981) to refer to this kind of breaking down of the opposition between signifier and signified. 'To reduce the signifier to a signified and declare that this is what the signifier means is to privilege the signified over the signifier. But Derrida insists that "every signified is also in the position of a signifier"' (Adams, 1992, p. 236). The refugees' experiences and their expression of their experiences are interrelated; the one constructs the other and both co-construct themselves.

Deconstruction asserts that

> any given body of statements, whether in everyday conversation or a scientific paper, depends on a number of other bodies of statements, some of which carry deeply entrenched convictions and explanatory schemas fundamental to the dominant form of making sense of the world at any particular period in a culture. Deconstruction retraces the system of 'dependencies' of a discourse. At the same time, it also has a positive foundation, in that it reconstructs a history which accounts for how a discourse or practice emerged, for the conditions of its emergence and constitution (discursive, material and historical) and for how it comes to be what it is at the present.
>
> (Henriques et al, 1984, p. 104)

Against this background, one cannot possibly see the role of the interpreter as that of a mere translating software, a faceless device. The interpreter's presence colours therapy inexorably and instead of trying to ignore or minimise his/her impact, we may as well endeavour to address it.

Therefore, the therapist can use the presence of the interpreter creatively in order to contribute to the deconstruction of the process of therapy itself. This can be done when the therapist avoids the trap of looking only for the perfect translation but also becomes attuned to the manner in which all three protagonists interact in therapy. Each one of them is affected by the presence of the other two, and instead of fighting against the effects of this, it may well be advised to acknowledge it as a potential beneficial additional source of information in therapy. Each one of them, as dramatis personae of this drama, has his or her own role to play. Thus, the therapeutic system consists of three parties and not only of two.

Co-therapists with a difference

During a recent piece of research (Papadopoulos, 1996b, 1998, 1999a; Papadopoulos and Hildebrand, 1997), with a colleague from the Tavistock Clinic (Judy Hildebrand), we interviewed families of Bosnian ex-camp prisoners who were asylum seekers in the UK. The unusual feature of this research was the fact that although both of us were experienced therapists, only one of us spoke the language of these families; as a result, as a team we performed two roles – that of interpreting and that of maintaining therapeutic contact. I was at the same time an interpreter, an interviewer and a therapist and Judy was the last two but not an interpreter. In this way, I had the unique experience of observing the therapeutic process (as an interpreter) as well as being part of it.

> On many occasions, Judy's role was comparable to that of a reflecting team in so far as she was one step removed from the direct conversation. When painful material emerged and one of us became too involved in their narrative, the other could maintain a more systemic role, keeping in mind the whole family system.
>
> (Papadopoulos and Hildebrand, 1997, p.222)

Overall, we found that there are positive and negative implications of the differences in our roles as co-therapists: on the positive side, we were enabled to split the functions and each one to concentrate on different aspects of the task (i.e. information gathering and empathetic listening); whereas on the negative side, the need for translation often slowed and de-intensified the pace of their narrative. What was also interesting was that we often realised (during our discussions at the end of each session) that we had honed in on different facets of the family story; invariably, this was directly connected with the different roles we played during the session. This does not mean that the one of us was right and the other was wrong; on the contrary, the stereoscopic perspective on the session which emerged enabled us to deconstruct the therapeutic process and understand more fully our positions in it, too.

Speaking their language, I was often put in a position where I felt extremely close to these Bosnian families and at a distance from my co-therapist who, then, seemed to me during the session 'not to understand'. This identification with the families made me realise

how difficult it must be for interpreters who do not possess therapeutic understanding and skills and who inevitably feel compelled
to take sides. In our case, Judy and I were able to discuss together
after each session all our observations and feelings and these
discussions invariably threw light on the sessions in ways that,
ordinarily, neither of us on our own would have been able to
access.

A therapist–interpreter faces many dilemmas. Occasionally I
experienced a particularly difficult dilemma, known in the literature: 'Sometimes, the client places the interpreter in a difficult
situation, by telling him something and then asking him not to
tell the therapist' (van der Veer, 1998, p.82). In most cases, my
response was to assure the families that I would not mention what
they had told me during the session but, since Judy and I were
colleagues and we wanted to think together about them, I needed
to think whether discussing it with Judy at a later stage would have
been helpful to them. By and large, they seemed to find this an
acceptable response.

Occupying a dual position, as interpreter and co-therapist,
introduced a new dimension in my understanding of the manner in
which 'dominant discourses' affect the process of interpreting. One
of the insights I had was in relation to the differences between the
therapist and the interpreter that can develop in the course of even
one interview. More specifically, I became aware of a sense of
antagonism in me in relation to Judy when she was trying to follow
a certain line of questioning that I felt was inappropriate. During
our interview with one family, things unfolded in a way that Judy
assumed the role of the main therapist and I was operating as an
interpreter; at a certain time I began feeling uncomfortable when
Judy was pursuing a line of exploring the nature of the traumatic
experiences the family had suffered. I felt that her questions were
emphasising the pathological aspects of the family and I was
feeling uneasy because, according to my understanding, that particular family was one of the most resilient families of the group that
we were working with. I felt, at the time, that I was aware of the
reasons for being uncomfortable and it was not because I did not
want to hear again their bad experiences; they had already told me
on a previous occasion all about those experiences, when I had first
met them without Judy. I felt that I was uncomfortable because I
thought that Judy's questions were not allowing the family to
convey their resilient side and I was afraid that the family would be

sliding into a victim position. As it turned out, Judy's questions were not inappropriate and she managed to elicit useful information about the differences within the family about their perceptions of the father's predicament. Nevertheless, the point I wish to make here is that during that brief period my antagonism towards Judy affected the way I was translating. More specifically, listening later to the audio recording of the session, I became aware that I translated the mother's complaint about the family's 'problems' (due to the father's worrying behaviour) as 'difficulties'; moreover, my intonation was such that clearly underplayed the family's distress. I was not conscious at the time that I translated 'problem' as 'difficulty' and I was surprised to hear that later.

This example demonstrates that overarching dominant discourses and their interrelation govern not only the interpreters' and therapists' understanding of the refugee family but also affect the very way things are translated. In this example, I was afraid that Judy was operating from the dominant discourse of the Post-Traumatic Stress 'Disorder' and was ignoring the 'resilient' discourse. As a result, my own attempt at remedying what I misperceived as a one-sidedness created a worse distortion of the material. However, this is not the only type of distortion that occurs in these settings. I have often found that some interpreters, in their effort to be on equal terms with the mental health professionals (for whom they translate), tend to assume a medical or psychiatric discourse and unwittingly thus colour their translations accordingly.

On the life of language and the language of life

The relevant literature on interpreters has, correctly, emphasised issues pertaining to their personal and emotional involvement in the process of therapy. However, the subjugation of individual discourses by dominant discourses in the society at large is something that has not been explored sufficiently. As was mentioned above, the process of translation in these contexts is not limited to inter- and intra-lingual translation but also includes inter-semiotic translation. It is in this category of translation that we should include the transfer of meaning from one discourse to the other. However, in order to be able to do this, one first needs to become aware of their powerful presence and appreciate the manner in which they affect us. Then, we will need to find our way through the thorny area of how to address the influence of these dominant discourses. Needless to say, everybody would want to enable the subjugated discourses to take root and begin to flourish. However, this is not an easy task. In family therapy theory and practice there has been the idea that the therapist should diminish the power of the dominant discourse and increase the power of the subjugated one (e.g. White and Epston, 1991). This, of course implies that (a) there is only one such discourse and (b) that the therapist or the family members are aware of it. But is this the case? Surely, there is not only one subjugated discourse complete and ready to be discovered. Such a discourse is created, is moulded in the process of therapy. Moreover, the best way of describing this process is to say that it is co-created and co-construed by all participants in the process of therapy, i.e. the therapist, the interpreter, and all the members of the family; in addition, these interactions do not take place in a vacuum but within the various dominant discourses, which are at times complementary and at times conflicting. The main protagonists assume their identities by the selective process of emphasising certain similarities and differences among them in the context of the all-engulfing discourses which privilege one time sequence over another or give it a specific meaning. It is in this alchemical state of interactions that the 'tyranny of the post' tends to dominate, due to its power and simplicity.

In the example above, I was caught up in my own struggle between two discourses that I had consciously distinguished myself; but in doing so, in that particular instance, I ignored the possible discourses that the family could have co-constructed with us. I fell into the trap of feeling that I was advocating their own discourse (as it happened, in subsequent meetings they were able to begin to articulate their own complex discourses). Interpreters can easily fall prey to their own perceptions of what is appropriate and what is right even if these perceptions are consciously available to them.

It is indeed very difficult for all concerned to accept that the interpreters' presence as well as the translation they produce have a life of their own that needs to be respected and interacted with, rather than ignored or even condemned. According to their 'job description', they should just be offering the services of a good translating software and not be present as interacting human beings. Everything said above points to the limitations of this view.

The 'immigrant', that Anne Michaels' translator is likened with, is a palpable reality. The otherness cannot be tamed into a familiar predictability. Translating is dealing with the open otherness which we cannot eradicate completely, regardless of our wish to do so. Our keenness to understand too much in a logical and definitive way and to foreclose all anxiety often makes us follow, unwittingly, a given predominant discourse. This amounts to privileging the language of life over the life of language which creates an illusion of comfort. However, the cost of this comfort is to lose the risky openness that venturing into the life of language affords, along with all its freshness and potentiality for revitalisation.

Acknowledgement

I wish to acknowledge the assistance of Judy Hildebrand for the joint work we have been doing and for her generous contribution to the development of some of the ideas expressed here in relation to our research project.

References

Adams, M.V. (1992) 'Deconstructing philosophy and imaginal psychology: comparative perspectives on Jacques Derrida and James Hillman'. In R.P. Sugg (ed.), *Jungian Literary Criticism*. Evanston, IL: Northwestern University Press.

Andersen, T. (1987) 'The reflecting team: dialogue and meta-dialogue in clinical work'. *Family Process*, 26(2): 415–428.

Andersen, T. (1992) 'Reflections and reflecting with families'. In S. McNamee and K. Gergen (eds), *Therapy as Social Construction*. London: Sage.

Bateson, G. [1969] (1972) 'Double Bind 1969'. In G. Bateson (ed.), *Steps to an Ecology of Mind*. New York: Ballantine.

Bowlby, J. [1973] (1985) *Attachment and Loss. Volume 2. Separation, Anxiety and Anger*. London: Pelican Books.

Bowlby, J. (1988) *A Secure Base: Parent–Child Attachment and Healthy Human Development*. New York: Basic Books.

Bracken, P.J. (1998) 'Hidden agendas. Deconstructing Post-Traumatic Stress Disorder'. In P.J. Bracken and C. Petty (eds), *Rethinking the Trauma of War*. London: Free Association Books.

Bracken, P.J. and Petty, C. (1998) (eds) *Rethinking the Trauma of War*. London: Free Association Books.

Cheshire, N.M. (1975) *The Nature of Psychodynamic Interpretation*. London: John Wiley and Sons.

Dallos, R. (1997) *Interacting Stories. Narratives, Family Beliefs, and Therapy*. London: Karnac Books.

de Certeau, M. (1986) *Heterologies. Discourse on the Other*. Manchester: Manchester University Press.

Derrida, J. (1978) *Writing and Difference*. Chicago: Chicago University Press.

Derrida, J. (1981) *Dissemination*. Chicago: Chicago University Press.

Edelson, M. (1975) *Language and Interpretation in Psychoanalysis*. New Haven: Yale University Press.

Felman, S. and Laub, D. (1992) *Testimony. Crises of Witnessing in Literature, Psychoanalysis and History*. London: Routledge.

Flanders, S. (1993) (ed.) *The Dream Discourse Today*. London: Routledge.

Friedman, M. and Jaranson, J. (1994) 'The applicability of the PTSD concept to refugees'. In A.J. Marsella, T. Borneman, S. Ekblad and J. Orley (eds), *Amidst Peril And Pain. The Mental Health And Social Well-Being Of The World's Refugees*. Washington, DC: American Psychological Association, pp. 207–228.

Fromm, E. (1951) *The Forgotten Language*. New York: Grove Press.

Henriques, J., Hollway, W., Urwin, C., Venn, C. and Walkerdine, P. (eds) (1984). *Changing the Subject. Psychology, Social Regulation and Subjectivity*. London: Methuen.

Ignatieff, M. (1999) *The Warrior's Honor. Ethnic War and the Modern Conscience*. London: Vintage.

Jakobson, R. (1971) 'On linguistic aspects of translation'. In *Selected Writings, Volume 2, Word and Language*, 260–266. The Hague: Mouton.

Kugler, P. (1982) *The Alchemy of Discourse. An Archetypal Approach to Language*. London: Associated University Presses.

Maffei, G. (1986) *I Linguaggi della Psihe*. Milano: Bompiani.

Mahony, P. (1987) *Psychoanalysis and Discourse*. London: Tavistock Publications.

Marsella, A.J., Friedman M.J. and Huland Spain, E. (1996a) 'Ethnocultural aspects of PTSD: an overview and issues and research directions'. In A.J. Marsella, M.J. Friedman, E.T. Gerrity and R. Scurfield (eds), *Ethnocultural Aspects of Post-traumatic Stress Disorder. Issues, Research, and Clinical Applications*. Washington, DC: American Psychological Association.

Marsella, A.J., Friedman, M.J., Gerrity, E.T. and Scurfield, R.M. (1996b) 'Ethnocultural aspects of PTSD: Some closing thoughts'. In A.J. Marsella, M.J. Friedman, E.T. Gerrity and R. Scurfield (eds), *Ethnocultural Aspects of Post-traumatic Stress Disorder. Issues, Research, and Clinical Applications*. Washington, DC: American Psychological Association.

Michaels, A. (1998) *Fugitive Pieces*. London: Bloomsbury.

Muller, J.P. (1996) *Beyond the Psychoanalytic Dyad. Developmental Semiotics in Freud, Peirce and Lacan*. London: Routledge.

Ogden, C.K. and Richards, I.A. [1923] (1949) *The Meaning of Meaning. A Study of the Influence of Language upon Thought and of the Science of Symbolism*. London: Routledge and Kegan Paul.

Papadopoulos, R. (1996a) 'Archetypal family therapy: developing a

Jungian approach to working with families'. In L. Dodson and T. Gibson (eds), *Psyche and Family*. Wilmette, IL: Chiron.

Papadopoulos, R.K. (1996b) 'Therapeutic presence and witnessing'. *The Tavistock Gazette*, (Autumn), 61–65.

Papadopoulos, R.K. (1997) 'Individual identity and collective narratives of conflict'. *Harvest: Journal for Jungian Studies*, 43(2): 7–26.

Papadopoulos, R.K. (1998) 'Destructiveness, atrocities and healing: epistemological and clinical reflections'. *The Journal of Analytical Psychology*, 43(4): 455–477.

Papadopoulos, R.K. (1999a) 'Working with families of Bosnian medical evacuees: therapeutic dilemmas'. *Clinical Child Psychology and Psychiatry*, 4(1): 107–120.

Papadopoulos, R.K. (1999b) 'Storied community as secure base'. *The British Journal of Psychotherapy*.

Papadopoulos, R.K. and Hildebrand, J. (1997) 'Is home where the heart is? Narratives of oppositional discourses in refugee families'. In R.K. Papadopoulos and J. Byng-Hall (eds), *Multiple Voices; Narrative in Systemic Family Psychotherapy*. London: Duckworth.

Papp, P. (1980) 'The Greek chorus and other techniques in family therapy'. *Family Process*, 19(1): 45–58.

Pentz-Moller, V., Bentsen, E.M., Hermansen, A., Knudsen, I.H. and Pentz-Moller, V. (1988) *Interpretation in the Rehabilitation of Torture Victims at the RCT*. Copenhagen: The International Research and Rehabilitation Centre for Torture Victims.

Putsch, R.W. (1985) 'Cross-cultural communication. The special case of interpreters in health care'. *Journal of the American Medical Association*, 254: 3344–3348.

Richman, N. (1998) 'Looking before and after: refugees and asylum seekers in the West'. In P.J. Bracken and C. Petty (eds), *Rethinking the Trauma of War*. London: Free Association Books.

Rimmon-Kenan, S. (1987) (ed.) *Discourse in Psychoanalysis and Literature*. London: Methuen.

Sabin, J.E. (1975) 'Translating despair'. *American Journal of Psychiatry*, 132: 197–199.

Siegelman, E.Y. (1990) *Metaphor and Meaning in Psychotherapy*. London: The Guilford Press.

Steiner, G. (1975) *After Babel. Aspects of Language and Translation*. Oxford: Oxford University Press.

van der Veer, G. (1998) *Counselling and Therapy with Refugees and Victims of Trauma. Psychological Problems of Victims of War, Torture and Repression*. Chichester: John Wiley and Sons, (second edition).

White, M. and Epston, D. (1991) *Narrative Means to Therapeutic Ends*. New York: W.W. Norton.

Chapter 16

Concluding comments

Rachel Tribe and Hitesh Raval

The editors have enjoyed the collaboration with the authors who have made valuable contributions to this book in what is an under reported yet important area of work. The authors have brought their perspectives on this work from a number of different service provision contexts and professional roles, such as having worked as interpreters, managing an interpreter's service, to clinicians who are working with interpreters.

Many health care service providers will face a continued need to utilise interpreters in order to meet the language and health care needs of ethnic minority service users who require the help of an interpreter. The chapters in this book have highlighted important areas that need further consideration and development.

The importance of training of interpreters and clinicians for both interpreters and clinicians has been highlighted by most of the authors. There remains a clear need for the provision of quality accredited training programs for interpreters in Britain, and this is likely to be the case in many other countries. There also remains a great degree of variability with regards to what such training provision should consist of and the types of skills that need to be developed for interpreters through such training. The training provision for clinicians remains largely unattended to, and this is likely to stay unaltered unless there are mandatory requirements for clinicians to develop their skills in being able to work more effectively with interpreters. Quality training that is provided at the highest standard is very much needed in order to minimise the patchy and variable training that is currently carried out. Issues related to recognising the professional status of interpreters, the provision of adequate management and career structures, and employment protection and the employment rights of interpreters also need urgent attention.

The authors have also brought their clinical experience to bear in the respective chapters. The wealth of experience of working with interpreters is reflected in many of the chapters. What comes through strongly is the need to make time to develop a working alliance between the interpreter and clinician. Ideally, where services are meeting the needs of large enough sections of the community needing an interpreter speaking a particular language or dialect, one would hope that this need would be met by employing an interpreter or bilingual worker specifically for that service. This model of employing interpreters has many advantages such as increasing the consistency, skills base, and familiarity of the work for both the interpreter and clinician. Where this is not possible or practical, it is still important to ensure that the same interpreter is available for the work with a given service user, as this increases the likelihood of engagement, containment, trust, continuity, and consistency for all the parties concerned.

Several authors have suggested models or frameworks for developing the clinical practice with interpreters. First, all the models have placed the emphasis on the importance of taking into account the personhood of the interpreter. As much as we would like it, interpreters cannot be expected to work as if they were a 'mouth piece' without their own feelings, views and opinions. Whilst a level of impartiality is required in therapeutic work, it is equally important that there is time made available to reflect on the emotional impact of carrying out therapeutic work with service users. This is needed for both the interpreter and the clinician. Time for briefing, de-briefing, and discussion is important in this area of work. Equally important is the provision of clinical supervision and effective management structures for interpreters. Systemic and psychoanalytic models of therapy have been used by some of the authors in helping us think about the role conflicts that can arise, and how emotional factors can have a direct impact on the way in which working or therapeutic alliances are formed in this three-way relationship. Ways to develop good practice have been suggested by many of the authors.

Different service contexts and user groups bring with them shared as well as unique mental health needs, and present different challenges to the service provider and interpreter. The chapters in this book have touched on shared issues, as well as particular concerns of service users, in describing the work taking place in a variety of heath care settings, and with different community populations. The issues and needs for established community groups, whilst sharing many similarities with regards to equity, discrimination, and access to services, are also very different in many other ways to the issues being faced by many refugee service users. What comes across for the chapters describing the work within the refugee context is the different order of life experiences and trauma that have been experienced by many of the refugee service users. This work brings into play a different dimension where interpreters need careful and much needed support, particularly if interpreters are to be protected from further personal traumatisation by the virtue of carrying out a piece of work with a traumatised service user.

What is also evident from the contributions to this book is that language, culture, and meaning are interconnected in rich and complex ways. Life is lived in language and language brings life to the lived experience. Translation and interpretation are required at numerous levels if a shared understanding of the meaning behind a lived experience is going to be conveyed in a helpful way. For this to happen the notion of a 'literal or verbatim' translation has to be abandoned. A lot of hard intricate work is required to render a translation in a meaningful and understandable way. Clinicians often undervalue the skills that are required of an interpreter in being able to carry out this complex task. Interpreters are often required to provide a culturally contextualised translation for it to have any relevance for the clinician or service user. The process of negotiating a shared understanding of the problem, and a jointly agreed plan of action in order to alleviate the problem, is both a subtle and complex one. For it to happen naturally and effectively, the roles taken on by an interpreter have to be varied.

Several of the authors in this book have made a case for enabling interpreters to take on a broader role in the work that goes beyond their role as translators. Interpreters play a vital role as bilingual or link-workers, as advocates, as cultural consultants or intermediaries, and as conciliators. Regular opportunities for joint working can increase the level of confidence and willingness of the clinician to encourage the interpreter in taking on a broader role in the work. At the same time it is important to note that interpreters should not be set tasks that go beyond their level of skill, experience and competence.

Complex co-working and relationship issues have to be negotiated by the interpreter, clinician and the service user if this three-way relationship is going to work well. These relationships have the potential to quickly become explosive and break down, further increasing the reluctance of many service users (and interpreters) to become involved with mental health providers. The likelihood of miscommunication and misunderstanding is high when people who do not know each other are coming together for the first time. Some of these difficulties can only be resolved if interpreters are employed on a permanent basis within a particular service provider setting, or they have the opportunity to work on a reasonably regular basis with clinicians from the same work setting.

It is the hope of the contributors in this book that the reader has found the chapters helpful and stimulating in thinking about and in being able to carry out work with interpreters. Another hope is that this book will open up a much broader dialogue of this important area of work, where to date so little has been written and where minimal research has been carried out, which could help towards improving clinical practice.

Index

abuse 178–9
accreditation 13, 20, 22; in UK 25
acquiescence effect 170
advice giving 48–9
advocacy 18, 19, 30–1, 34, 42, 49, 70, 102, 115, 192–3, 208, 258
age, issues of 63, 106–7, 122, 222, 195, 234
agencies 57, 62, 80–3, 102; accountability 60; best practice guidelines 60; daily life in 77–91; induction courses 60; multiple 108
Albania and Albanians 88
alienation and marginalisation 164–5
alliances, inappropriate 159
Amato, R. 135
America see United States of America
Amharic language 85–6
Arabic interpreters 84
Asian families, bilingualism in 168
asylum seekers 58, 199, 201, 212, 220, 249; Bosnian 249–51; psychological effect on 200, 202; vulnerability of 201
Audit Commission (UK), recommendation by 11
Australia 11, 65, 145, 202, 209; legislation in 11; New South Wales 42–3, 55
Ayres, W. 160

Baker, R. 220
Balint Groups 235
Balint, M. 235
Bangladesh and Bangladeshis 136–41, 149, 151, 155–7, 159–61, 165
Bateson, G. 183
Benefits Agency, UK 81, 87
Bengal and Bengalis 156
Bengali language 160; speakers of 155
bias effect 104
bilingualism 13, 22
booking interpreters 62–4; specificity of requirements 90
Bradford, UK 154
Britain see United Kingdom

Cambodia and Cambodians 203
Canada 9, 11; legislation in 11
Cantonese interpreter 88
career issues concerning interpreters: alternative employment 118; availability 82–3, 102, 114; booking 62–4; dissatisfaction 117; fees 24; job skills 109–11; lack of identity 2; length of service 107–8, 118; need for 11–13, 69–70, 256; perspectives on profession 16, 92–8, **104–5**; remuneration 114, 117; satisfaction **106**; travel 102, 114; turnover 82; value of 207–8; volunteers 13, 208

carers 171; Japanese 17; social
   pressures upon 169–70
case histories, importance of 66
case studies 37–8, 43–4, 139,
   141–4, 153, 159–64, 169–70, 189,
   191–2, 194, 200–1, 205
Cheatham, H. 125
Children Act (1989) UK, racial
   requirements of 155
children: abuse of 20; (sexual 210);
   experiences of 159–61
Chinese communities 155
circularity 193
class system 185, 222, 234; effect of
   33, 78
clients: choices by 233; deaf 2, 140;
   family social history of 173;
   gender of 174; matching 117; re-
   empowerment of 233; see also
   service users
clinicians: attitude problems of
   112–13; feelings about
   interpretation services 100–1;
   (detachment 21, 100, 159);
   (frustration 21, 146); (hostility
   and mistrust 49, 57, 136);
   (powerlessness 21); guidelines for
   61–8, 95–6; power imbalance
   with service user 33, 49, 57;
   problems experienced by 19–20,
   49, 100–1; training 50, 110; (lack
   of 20, 187); treatment approaches
   of 95–6; working with
   interpreters 64, 135–150; see also
   doctors; health professionals;
   practitioners
cognitive ability in pwld 175
cognitive bias 170
communication: ambiguity in 189;
   concepts of health and illness 34;
   cosmopolitan 149; cross-cultural
   40; effective 34–5, 69; language
   in 34; non-verbal 17, 40–1, 47,
   186; (aggression/self harm 171);
   process of translation 15–17, 34;
   style of 34, 40; theory 135
communities, storied 244
community: advocate 18; helpers
   72; interpreting 87

conciliator 18
confidentiality 21, 31, 33, 72, 175;
   training in 59
Congo 207
consultations: bilingual 46–8;
   guidelines for 46–8; medical
   30–53; (problems with
   terminology 30); see also
   interviews; meetings
context, significance of 128–30, 183
Corsellis, A. 12, 14–15
cost of services 118–19
countertransference 204, 235
Croatia and Croatians 85
Cronen, V. 126
culture and cultural issues 65–6, 71,
   92, 140, 156, 175, 185–7, 210–11,
   219, 224, 227, 233; cultural
   advisor 157; cultural beliefs 38;
   (and mental health **39**); cultural
   bereavement 203; cultural broker
   17, 34, 56, 93, 99, 102, 122,
   127–8, 234; cultural consultant 3,
   17, 56, 122, 172, 193, 258;
   cultural differences 78; (etiquette
   111); cultural identity 122;
   cultural information, need for
   72–3; cultural insensitivity 9;
   cultural perspectives 24; cultural
   sensitivity 117; cultural types:
   (emotional 40); (stoical 40);
   cultural values, irreconcilable 31;
   defined 122; multi-cultural issues
   122; (counselling 125);
   (frameworks 124–5); (theories,
   significance of 130–1); (therapy
   (MCT) 125); (movement 207);
   web of meanings 122

decipherment, interpretative 242
deconstruction 248
Denmark 204, 211
dependency, mutual 222
depression, concept of 38
Derrida, J. 248
diagnoses, western 11
Diagnostic Statistical Manual
   (DSM-IV) 204
dialect 62, 92

Diploma in Public Service Interpreting (DPSI) 55
discourse: dominant 251–2; (and interpretation 250–1); subjugated 252
discrimination 56
doctors: perceived omnipotence of 33; relationship with service user 32–5, 41–2; (power and control in 32–4); *see also* clinicians; health professionals; practitioners
dyad 211; synapse 242, 247

Education Departments (UK) 155
embarrassment, difficulties caused by 98, 118
emotion and emotional issues concerning interpreters 113, 129–30, 142–5, 235–6; distress 201–2; embarrassment 98, 118; ethical guidelines for 23–4; expression 41; impacts 158; impartiality and neutrality 64, 96–7; personal experience 101–6; problems 205; professional detachment 89; sensitive information and 57–8; sensitivity of 62–3; vocabulary 174–5
employment rights 257
English language 209
Eritrea 85–6
Essential Interpreters and Translators International (EITI) 62, 68
ethics 3, 31; ethical considerations 59; (impartiality and neutrality 64, 96–7); (professional detachment 89); (self-determination 24, 31); (sensitive information 57–8); ethical guidelines 23–4; (North American 23)
Ethiopia and Ethiopians 85–6
ethnicity 122, 185, 187, 222, 234, 245
Eurocentric psychological models 220
Exceptional Leave to Remain status (UK) 199

exile 229; experience of 232; process of 220

Falicov, C.J. 122–4, 130
families: ecological context 123; migration and acculturation context 123; life-cycle 123; organisation 123; rules and customs in 161
Farooq, S. 139–40, 145
frameworks: cross-cultural 128; ecological 122–4, 128; theoretical 122–34; usefulness to clinicians 128
France 207
Freed, A. 17, 145, 147
French language 207; speakers of 224–5

Geertz, C. 122
gender, issues of 63, 78–9, 107, 122, 185, 222, 234, 245; problems caused by 19
Grasska, M.A. 187
guidelines for working with interpreters 61–8, 101; subject matter 62–3; booking procedure 62–4; (agencies' role 62); determination of language and dialect 62; future meetings 64; good practice **105**–106; support and supervision 59, 130, 235

Harvey, M. 139
Health Advisory Commission (UK) 11
health and illness, concepts of 34, 38–40
health authorities: career development in 74–5; dedicated sessions 73–4; health promotion by 74; home support 73; language support services 73; locality-based services 73; recruitment by 74–5; service specifications 73; specialist services 74; staff retention 74–5; training, possibility of 57

health care services: discrepancies
in provision of information 69;
language provision in 69–76
health pluralism 206
health professionals: concerns
about working with interpreters
48–9; post-consultation meetings
48; pre-consultation meeting
45–6; training implications 50;
see also clinicians; doctors;
practitioners
help-seeking behaviour 205–7
Henriques, J. 248
high monitors 231
Hildebrand, J. 249–51
Home Office, UK 199
hostility 49, 57, 101, 136; difficulty
of translating 163
human rights 220, 230; abuses of
221–2, 227; political stance 222

illness and health, concepts of 34,
38–40
immigrants 140, 152–4; Asian
population, UK 80–1;
expectations of 152
immigration 162, 165; patterns of
156
Immigration and Asylum Bill
(1999), UK 200
income tax, UK 86; Pay As You
Earn (PAYE) 86
information, sensitive 57–8
informed consent 19, 33
inhibition effect 105, 108
Institute of Linguists, UK 55;
accredited training courses 55;
DPSI 55
interpretation: courses in 55;
(Antipodes 55); (Australia 55);
cultural 186; digital 186; distortion
of 36, 48–9; levels of 185–6;
linguistic 185; metaphorical
185–6; resolving problems with
49–50; triangle 146–7
interpreters, career issues
concerning: alternative
employment 118; availability
82–3, 102, 114; booking 62–4;

dissatisfaction 117; fees 24; job
skills 109–11; lack of identity 2;
length of service 107–8, 118; need
for 11–13, 69–70, 256;
perspectives on profession 16,
92–8, **104–5**; remuneration 114,
117; satisfaction **106**; travel 102,
114; turnover 82; value of 207–8;
volunteers 13, 208
interpreters, emotional issues
concerning 113, 129–30, 142–5,
235–6; distress 201–2;
embarrassment 98, 118; ethical
guidelines for 23–4; expression
41; impacts 158; impartiality and
neutrality 64, 96–7; personal
experience 101–6; problems 205;
professional detachment 89;
sensitive information and 57–8;
sensitivity of 62–3; vocabulary
174–5
interpreters, problems in working
with 8–29, 48–9, 209; conflicts
14–16; detachment 100;
difficulties **104–5**, 111–14;
distortion of translation 48, 146;
embarrassment 100; extrinsic 187;
frustration 101; health worker
concerns 48–9, 209; hostility 101;
individual 'agenda' 49; intrinsic
187; issues in working with 8–29,
48–9, 209; negative emotional
states 100; negative emphasis 187;
power struggles 101; professional
jealousy 101; suspicion 100;
tension 49, 96; unhelpful
coalitions 100
interpreters, professional issues
concerning: accreditation 13, 22;
age 106–7, 195; demography **103**,
166–8; education 107;
empowerment 188; experience
99–121; gender 107; legal
requirements 13; professionalism
147–8; qualifications 107, 157;
role boundaries 137–9, 211; self
confidence 3, 164; skills 14, 16,
22, 79, 93, 96; status 2, 20, 22, 83,
158, 256

interpreters, the roles of 11, 16,
17–20, 30, 70–1, 74–5, 93,
99–121, 130, 132, 151–67, 186,
207–8, 248; advice giver 48–9;
advocate 18, 19, 30–1, 34, 49, 70,
102, 115, 192–3, 208, 258;
bilingual worker 18, 30, 35, 70,
192; conciliator 18; counsellor 74;
cultural advisor/consultant 17,
19, 56, 122, 157, 172, 193, 258;
cultural broker 17, 19, 34, 56, 93,
99, 102, 122, 127–8, 175, 234;
health advisor 70, 74; link worker
18, 56, 70, 208; role model 211;
specialist services 72, 74; (adult
mental health 182–97, 208–9);
(child mental health 151–67);
(medical consultations 30–5);
(primary care 72); translator 17,
30, 34, 102–6, 128
interpreters, working effectively
with 12, 45, 64, 135–50, 187–8,
209–10, 259; active participation
190–1, 195–6; appropriateness
for subject 62–3; continuity and
trust 97–8, 113–14, 257;
flexibility and freedom of
determination 165; guidelines
61–8, 101; good practice
105–106; health worker concerns
48–9; positive use of 139–42;
settings 55; style of 226–30;
support and supervision 59, 130,
235; theoretical frameworks for
108, 122–34
interpreting: agencies *see* agencies;
context of 188–90; criteria for 93;
models of 3, 55, 75–6; with
refugees 238–55; service, daily
life in 77–91; simultaneous 94;
techniques of 93–4; telephone 75,
81–2
interventions: contextual 124;
individual 124
interviews: conducted across social
environments 170; context of
132; *see also* consultations;
meetings

Japanese adults, as carers 17
job: confidence 108; dissatisfaction
117; satisfaction 108; skills
109–11

Kaufert, J.M. 24, 36, 38, 126–7,
131
Kenya 90
Kline, F. 21
knowledge, contextual 185–6
Koolage, W.W. 36, 38
Kosovans and Kosovo 88

language 92, 122, 219, 222, 245,
251–3; as basis of meaning
183–4; and cultural context,
interplay 184; gaps 10;
interchangeability, lack of 209;
misunderstanding as response
avoidance 175; support provider,
roles of 74; support services,
lack of 71–73; and translation
35–8; variability of
expressiveness 11
language, clarity of: avoidance of
jargon 67; avoidance of proverbs
and sayings 66; use of
dictionaries 60; use of first person
144; literal sense 66;
standardisation 60; variation 66,
79
languages: Amharic 85–6; Bengali
160; English 209; French 207;
Linghala 225; Mirpuri 139,
145; Spanish 21; Swahili 90;
Sylheti 151–3, 157, 161; Tigrinya
85–6
learning disabilities, people with
(pwld) 168–81; counselling of
179; interpretation services for
168–81; linguistic competence of
171; mental health problems and
170; parental attitudes to 168;
proportion within population
168
legal issues 105
Likert Scale **106**
Linghala language 225
link worker 18

literacy levels 156
locality-based services 73
logistics 3
London Open College Network
(LOCN) 56; course for
interpreters 56; (core units 56)
London, UK 138; East London
151, 155; Inner London 155;
Tower Hamlets 140

McFarland, T. 187
Marcos, L.R. 16, 18, 36
marriage problems 20, 105,
108
meaning: context dependent 126;
lack of shared system 137;
makers of 135–50; making
together 148–9; shared 148;
significance of 131–2
Meaning of Meaning, The (1923)
241
meetings 3, 31–2, 65–7; bilingual
46–8; breaks during 67, 94;
brevity, importance of 42, 94;
complexity of 31–2; cost-
effectiveness 70; effective
communication in 34–5;
(technical jargon in 67);
(dictionaries, use during 60);
goals 178; guidelines for
good practice 46–8, 95;
importance of introductions 66;
positive behaviours 35; post
session discussion/debriefing 48,
67–8, 98, 193–4, 196, 257;
preparatory discussion/briefing
45–6, 65–6, 94–6, 98, 178, 188,
190, 192–3, 196, 257; procedures
during 66–7, 193; roles of
participants in 31, 35; same
language 31–2; see also
consultations; interviews
mental disorders, reactive 203
mental health 205–7; adult 182–97;
(working with interpreters in
182–97); care provision,
restricted access to 9;
categorisation of refugees 202–4;
child 151–67; (role of the

interpreter in 151–67); (team in
context 154–7); and cultural
beliefs 39; language of 207;
practitioners in 13–15; sources of
help 205–7; translation
difficulties within 79
Mental Health Act (UK) 58
Michaels, A. 238, 252
migrant communities in New South
Wales, study of 24–3
Milan group 196
Milan systemic approach:
application of 192–5
Miller, G. 135
minority ethnic groups 221;
bilingual competence within 168;
culture 165; mental health care,
provision of 9–10; monitoring
and level of need 80; (censuses
and surveys 80)
Mirpuri language 139, 145
misdiagnosis 209
misinterpretation 36
models: advocacy m. 211;
alternative m. 148–9;
biopsychosocial m. 42; ecological
m. 123; explanatory m. 127;
inclusive m. 191; interpreting, m.
of 75–6, 211; linguistic m. 75,
211; mutual participation m. 33;
need for flexibility in use of 76;
professional team member m.
211; psycho-biomedical m.
126–8; psychological m. 174;
service provider team m. 75;
service user m. 75–6; theoretical
m. 123; (dealing with meaning
126–8)
moral stance 222

Nafsiyat Intercultural Centre,
London, UK 212
narratives: personal and
professional 191–2; post
traumatic 243–4
National Health Service, UK 55,
70, 208
national insurance contributions,
UK 86

Nationality, Immigration and
    Asylum Bill (2002), UK 200
nationality issues 63
normalisation 169
Norway 201–2

Ogden, C.K. 241
Open College Federation, UK 56

Pakistani communities 155
Papadopoulos, R. 249–51
parents: perceptions of health
    service 151; understanding
    concerns of 161–4; benefits of
    empowerment 151
partnership approach 33;
    misinterpretation of 42
Pearce, W. 135, 137, 149, 186–7
personal social network approach
    171–3; core phases 177; key
    attributes 172
personhood of interpreter 129, 136,
    138, 149
politics and political issues 85,
    88–9, 105, 111, 156, 219, 222,
    224, 227, 234; persecution 230;
    power, loss of 219–21; views 210;
    violence 220
'post office' model of
    communication 135, 148;
    interpreter as 'postman' 135–9
Post Traumatic Stress Disorder
    (PTSD) 203–4, 243–4, 251
post-structuralists 248
potential shared attributes 172,
    173–4; common specific training
    172; cultural stance 172, 175;
    emotional vocabulary 172,
    174–5; implications for clinical
    practice 177–9; professional
    training 172; religious affiliation
    172, 176; social history 172,
    173–4; syntax possession 172,
    176–7
power and empowerment 32–4, 56,
    147–8; imbalance 34, 49, 57, 148,
    187–8, 191, 224, 228–9;
    inappropriate 15; paradox of
    221; within triad 221–6

practice, clinical 3; no theoretical
    foundation for 8
practice, code of: desire for 117–18;
    for interpreters 37
practitioners: in mental health
    13–15; self-reflexivity of 185; see
    also doctors; clinicians; health
    professionals
presenting, clinical; somatic 206;
    medical 58; psychological 206
problems in working with
    interpreters 8–29, 48–9, 209;
    conflicts 14–16; detachment 100;
    difficulties 104–5, 111–14;
    distortion of translation 48, 146;
    embarrassment 100; extrinsic
    187; frustration 101; health
    worker concerns 48–9, 209;
    hostility 101; individual 'agenda'
    49; intrinsic 187; issues in
    working with 8–29, 48–9, 209;
    negative emotional states 100;
    negative emphasis 187; power
    struggles 101; professional
    jealousy 101; suspicion 100;
    tension 49, 96; unhelpful
    coalitions 100
professional boundaries 3;
    dilemmas 4
professional help: personal level
    123; political level 123; social
    level 123
professional issues concerning
    interpreters: accreditation 13, 22;
    age 106–7, 195; demography 103,
    166–8; education 107;
    empowerment 188; experience
    99–121; gender 107; legal
    requirements 13; professionalism
    147–8; qualifications 107, 157;
    role boundaries 137–9, 211; self
    confidence 3, 164; skills 14, 16,
    22, 79, 93, 96; status 2, 20, 22, 83,
    158, 256
psychiatric treatment,
    impossibility of effective
    therapy 139
psychiatrists, problems experienced
    by 21

psychology and psychological issues 105, 108; causes of ill health 39; cross-cultural 204; framework, influences on 123, language of 207; models 174; (problematisation of individuals 174); therapy 206; (relationship with culture 206–7); well being 179; (and service access 179)
PTSD 11
purchasing tools 73–5
Putsch, R.W. 24

qualifications in interpreting, lack of in UK 55
questions: leading 44; open 43; technique 170

race and culture: awareness 15; in clinical training 14
Race Relations Act, UK 155; funding for ethnic recruitment 155
racism 21, 40, 56–57, 162, 165, 177–8, 202, 204, 220, 229–30; institutional 9; overt 152; western health beliefs as a form of 57
Rack, P. 152
Raval, H. 142
refugees 4, 56, 80, 113, 115, 198–218, 208, 210, 218, 220, 229, 238–55; Cambodian 203; challenging the silence of 230–6; Chilean 202; community groups 212; Congolese 207; context, role of interpreters in 198–218; definition of 199; differences from migrants 198; disempowerment of 219–36; interpreting with 238–55; issues of trust 210–11; limited choice of self definition by language 225; and mental health 202–4; Middle Eastern 211; migration patterns to UK 198–200; Mozambican 202; multiplicity of 219–21; psychological problems 202–3; seeking asylum 199; service users 258; Somali 81; South East Asian

206; translating with 238–55; working with 210–12, 219–36
relationships: development of 3; doctor-service user 32–4
religion 63, 65–6, 78–9, 88–9, 92, 111, 122, 140, 156, 185–6, 210, 220, 222, 224, 227, 234, 245
Rennie, S. 139
République démocratique du Congo 207
resources, lack of 81
response avoidance 175
Richards, I.A. 241
Richardson, A. 169–70
Ritchie, J. 169–70
role of interpreters, the 11, 16, 17–20, 30, 70–1, 74–5, 93, 99–121, 130, 132, 151–67, 186, 207–8, 248; advice giver 48–9; advocate 18, 19, 30–1, 34, 49, 70, 102, 115, 192–3, 208, 258; bilingual worker 18, 30, 35, 70, 192; conciliator 18; counsellor 74; cultural advisor/consultant 17, 19, 56, 122, 157, 172, 193, 258; cultural broker 17, 19, 34, 56, 93, 99, 102, 122, 127–8, 175, 234; health advisor 70, 74; link worker 18, 56, 70, 208; role model 211; specialist services 72, 74; (adult mental health 182–97, 208–9); (child mental health 151–67); (medical consultations 30–5); (primary care 72); translator 17, 30, 34, 102–6, 128
role play and discussion 58–9
Roy, C.B. 17

self-injury 178
Serbia and Serbians 85
service: quality of 15; specifications 73–5
service delivery/provision 204; culturally appropriate 205; factors influencing 10; quality of 10; variations within UK 12
service providers, professional see doctors; clinicians; health professionals; practitioners

service users; centred model of interpreting 75; dialect 62; dissatisfaction 153; ethnic fit with interpreters 92; fluency 62; (first choice language(s) 62); inappropriate choice of translator 72; (friends and children 72); language gap 10, 70–2; need for information 72; perspective 100; pre-consultation meetings 46; relationships: (with doctor 32–3); (with interpreter 21); reluctance to use services 71; see also clients
sex and sexual issues 105, 108; sexual orientation 122
sign language, role of 17
signifier and signified 248
Smail, D, 123
social issues 105, 111; behaviour 41; constructionism 7; context assessment 170; role valorisation 169
Social Services Departments (UK) 155
social support 201–2
socio-economic situation 122
socio-political considerations 10
Solomon, M.Z. 23–4
Somali communities 155
South Africa 9
South Asian people in UK 40
Spanish-speaking clients 21
specialist interpreting services 72, 74; adult mental health 182–97, 208–9; child mental health 151–67; medical consultations 30–5; primary care 72
Speigal, J. 123
spiritual causal explanations 128–9
Steiner, G. 242
stigmas 206
stoicism 40–1
Sue, D.W. 125
support level 169
Swahili language 90
Sylhet, Bangladesh 149, 161
Sylheti language 151–3, 157, 161; speakers of 155

systemic social constructionist perspective 182; web of meanings 183–5

taboos 35, 42–5, 92, 111; fear of offence 43
task boundaries 58–9
Tavistock Clinic, UK 249
team working 142, 193; desirability of 115–16; relationships 164–5
telephone interpreting 245
terminology, need to learn 147
therapy and therapeutic issues 6, 211; context 221; details of 232; models; (Western 221); (neutrality of 221); interpreters as an aid to 139–40, 235; predictability as an aid to 231–2; process 245–6; relationships; (parents-therapist 162); (therapist-bilingual worker 162); system 193–4, 211; work 6, 20–3, 219; sessions see meetings
therapist: authoritarian 226; and interpreter, dilemmas of 250
Tigrinya language 85–6
time factors 111, 189
tone matching, importance of 97
torture 220, 228, 230–2; effect of 230–1
total body pain 39
training 3, 13–15, 50, 54–68, 82, 95, 99, 110, 118, 157, 256; at agency level 57; areas best included 14–15; in confidentiality 59; context dependent 13, 57; cross-cultural 15, 20; definition of modules 57; at health authority level 57; implications 50; lack of 20, 102, 187, 208; (restricted access to 56); not mandatory 8; model 148; modules 58–9; at national level 56–7; need for 118; place of 147–8; and qualifications 55–61, 107; and recruitment 82; seminars, need for 75; support during 14, 118

transference 21, 57, 211, 235
translation: aspects of 238–40; and
    communication, process of
    15–17; consecutive 35–6; defined
    240, 247; distortion of 16, 36;
    inappropriate 97; and
    interpretation, interrelationship
    of 240–2; lack of linguistic
    equivalence 36; and language
    35–8; with refugees 238–55;
    resemblance to psychotherapy
    243; simultaneous 35–6; types of
    241; (inter-lingual 241–2, 251);
    (inter-semiotic 241–2, 251);
    (intra-lingual 241–2, 251); (non-
    verbal 241); verbatim 3
translator 17; neutral mouthpiece
    18
trauma 122, 201, 204, 210, 243–4;
    dominant trauma discourse
    244; and life experiences 244;
    original 247; traumatisation,
    vicarious 235; traumatised service
    users 258; triple trauma
    paradigm 220
travel costs 87–8
triad 182, 185, 208, 211, 213;
    consensus within 130; interaction
    245; power relations within
    221–2, **223**–6; therapeutic 223
Tuckett, D. 31

United Kingdom 9, 55, 168–9,
    198–200, 202, 208, 220, 249;
    Immigration and Nationality
    Department 199; migration and
    refugees 198
United Nations Convention
    Relating to the Status of
    Refugees (1951) 199
United Nations Declaration of
    Human Rights (1948), Article 5
    220

United States of America (USA)
    202, 204, 206

videos, informational 74
Vietnamese communities 155

web of meanings within culture 122
welfare benefits 202
Westermeyer J. 225–226, 229
Wittgenstein, L. 136
workers: bicultural 211, 209;
    bilingual 18, 30, 56, 70–1, 154,
    157, 160–1, 190, 257;
    (containment by 163–4); (future
    development of 166);
    (recruitment of 157–9);
    (inappropriate use of staff as 12)
working effectively with
    interpreters 12, 45, 64, 135–50,
    187–8, 209–10, 259; active
    participation 190–1, 195–6;
    appropriateness for subject 62–3;
    continuity and trust 97–8,
    113–14, 257; flexibility and
    freedom of determination 165;
    guidelines 61–8, 101; good
    practice **105**–106; health worker
    concerns 48–9; positive use of
    139–42; settings 55; style of
    226–30; support and supervision
    59, 130, 235; theoretical
    frameworks for 108, 122–34
working practices, mutual 145–6
working style 226–30: amorphous
    226–7; colonial 229–30;
    constrictive 226; co-worker
    228–9; human rights workers
    227; judicial 227–8; team 142,
    193; (desirability of 115–16);
    (relationships 164–5); vague
    226–7

Zaire 207, 224

Index compiled by Lewis Derrick